ABSTRACT SYMMETRY
Geometric Coloring Book for Adults

175 Geometric Designs, Patterns and Shapes
to Color for Relaxing and Relieving Stress

ART THERAPY COLORING BOOK SERIES
[VOLUME FOUR]

THE MINDFUL WORD
www.themindfulword.org

Printed in the United States of America

ISBN 978-1-987869-42-2

Book design: Dew Media

The Mindful Word
701-1120 Finch Ave. W. #928
Toronto, Ontario
M3J 3H7, Canada

www.themindfulword.org

INTRODUCTION TO ART THERAPY

"Art is the meeting ground of the world inside and the world outside." - Elinor Ulman

As an artist, art therapist and mother I have been privileged to bear witness to the healing power of making art. I have experienced for myself the catharsis of becoming absorbed in a painting—my stress dissipating as I completely tune into the project at hand. As a therapist, I have seen clients make deep connections about themselves through exploring symbolism in their collage, painting and sculpture. I have watched my children become calmer and more focused while making crafts, drawing or scrapbooking.

By its very nature we intuitively know that art is healing and therapeutic—but why? Is it the process itself, the actual act of making art that soothes our nerves and settles our brains? Is it the freedom of expression it allows us? The metaphor and symbolism it can access from our unconscious minds? Or is it the pride and sense of accomplishment we take in the final product; the actual act of creating something that connects us to ourselves and the world on a deeper level? These questions form the basis for art therapy practice. And though art therapists acknowledge the artistic creations of their clients, the final product is not emphasized. Art therapy is concerned with the artistic process, symbolism and metaphors that are brought forth in the art.

Among art therapists a dichotomy exists as to why art therapy works. Is the creative process itself the therapy? Or does the artwork act as a form of communication between the client and the therapist? From my experience, art therapy functions as a combination of these two perspectives, facilitating both catharsis and therapeutic expression. The needs and abilities of the clients will often determine how the art process works and how the healing takes place. In some people the art will act to access the unconscious mind, uncovering new insights that can be discussed with the therapist. Some clients may have disabilities that create verbal challenges; for some it is too painful to talk about an "unspeakable" trauma or abuse. In these cases the art acts as a bridge, allowing clients to express themselves and tell their stories for the first time. In children, sculpting with clay may work effectively both as a process of cathartic release and an expression of difficult emotions. Art therapy is quickly able to get us in touch with our intuition and subconscious mind, cutting through over-thinking and emotional defenses that have built-up over the years.

A relatively new form of intervention, art therapy has been around as a profession since the 1940s. Since then, it has become recognized in the health profession as a powerful tool of self-expression and is often used interchangeably whenever psychotherapy is needed. Because of its non-threatening accessibility, art therapy is widely practiced as a therapy for people of all ages, backgrounds and abilities. It is used in a variety of settings with children, youth, veterans, adults, families and groups. From increasing self-awareness and well-being to empowerment, art therapy is an effective therapeutic approach for issues such as: bereavement and loss, depression and anxiety, trauma and abuse, chronic pain, anger, eating disorders and a variety of other issues. It can be used a primary form of therapy or an adjunct with other interventions. Art therapists have become integral to many treatment teams in hospitals, wellness clinics and schools.

A common concern for people when considering art therapy is that they have little to no experience in visual art. Although art therapists commonly have a background in the arts, clients need absolutely no expertise in art making. Art therapy is not concerned with how well someone draws or paints—or if they can at all. In fact, art therapists generally believe that trying to create art based on aesthetics in a session often blocks the therapeutic process. There are no mistakes or wrong ways of doing it. The therapist focuses on artistic expression and response, not the final product. For example, I have seen a client paint a very detailed picture and in the end completely cover the image in broad strokes of paint. Her reason for doing this was part of her therapeutic process—it was both symbolic and cathartic. In the end it didn't matter what her picture looked like—layers of red paint—but what did matter was how she was able to process this experience.

Art therapy sessions are easily adapted to the art modality the client feels most comfortable with such as painting, drawing or sculpture. Often the first few sessions may involve creating a collage. This activity provides an introduction to art-making for clients and starts to get them in touch with their creativity. From there the client may feel more at ease and want to experiment with other art media. Traditionally, art therapy utilized media such as paints, pastels, clay and pencils but increasingly art therapists are integrating other forms of artistic expression into their practice such as photography, video art, comic book creation and computer animation.

Although its roots are firmly based in psychoanalytic theory, art therapy is now finding its way in the areas of neuroscience, wellness, cognitive therapy and culturally sensitive practices. New approaches and research continue to reinforce that art therapy is a significantly beneficial form of intervention for a variety of people and complex issues. Inherently healing and life affirming, art therapy provides us with the tools to discover our own inner resources and strength.

- Catherine Gillespie-Lopes

"Expressive art therapy integrates all of the arts in a safe, non-judgmental setting to facilitate personal growth and healing. To use the arts expressively means going into our inner realms to discover feelings and to express them through visual art, movement, sound, writing or drama. This process fosters release, self-understanding, insight and awakens creativity and transpersonal states of consciousness." - Natalie Rogers

"The aim of art is to represent not the outward appearance of things, but their inward significance." – Aristotle

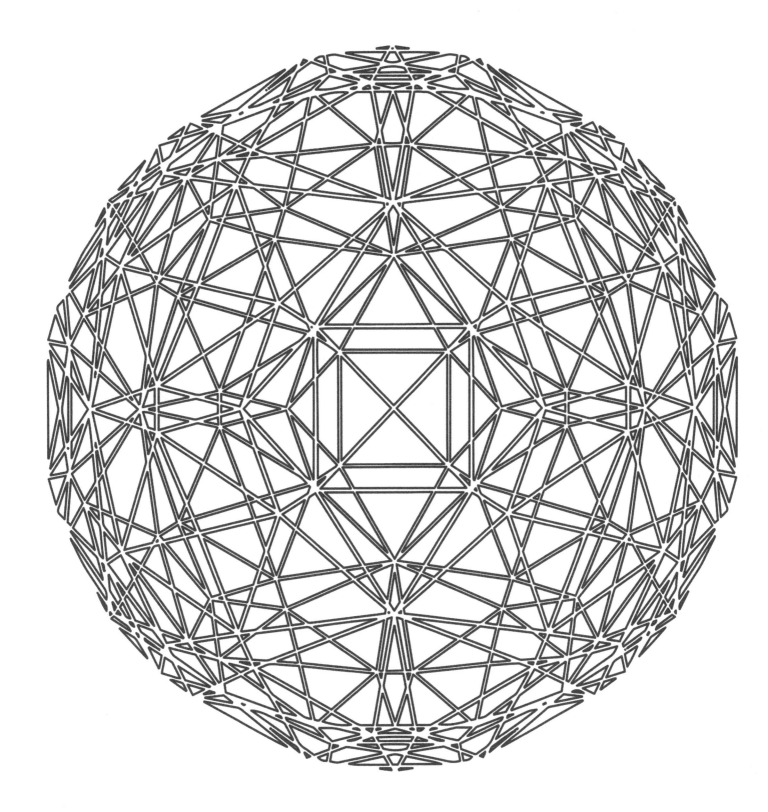

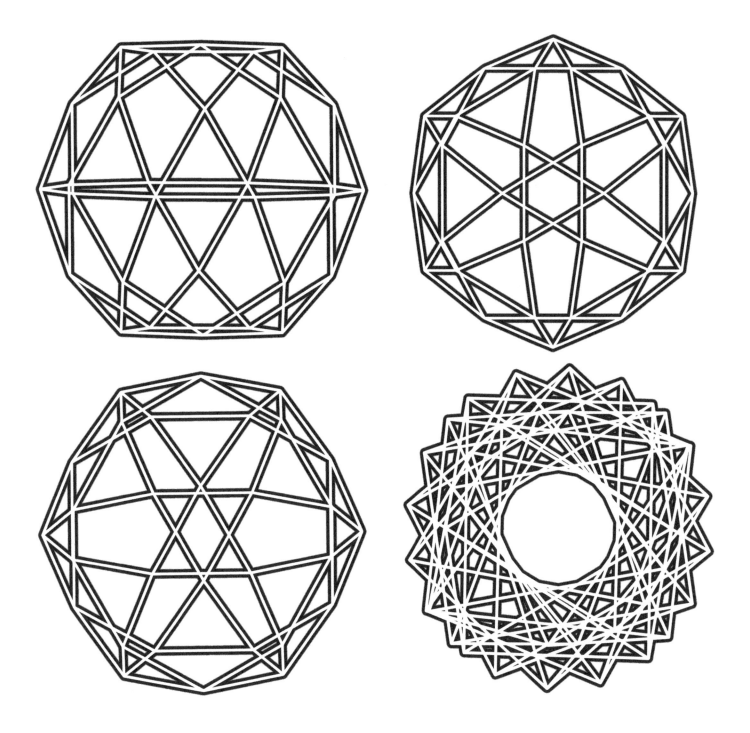

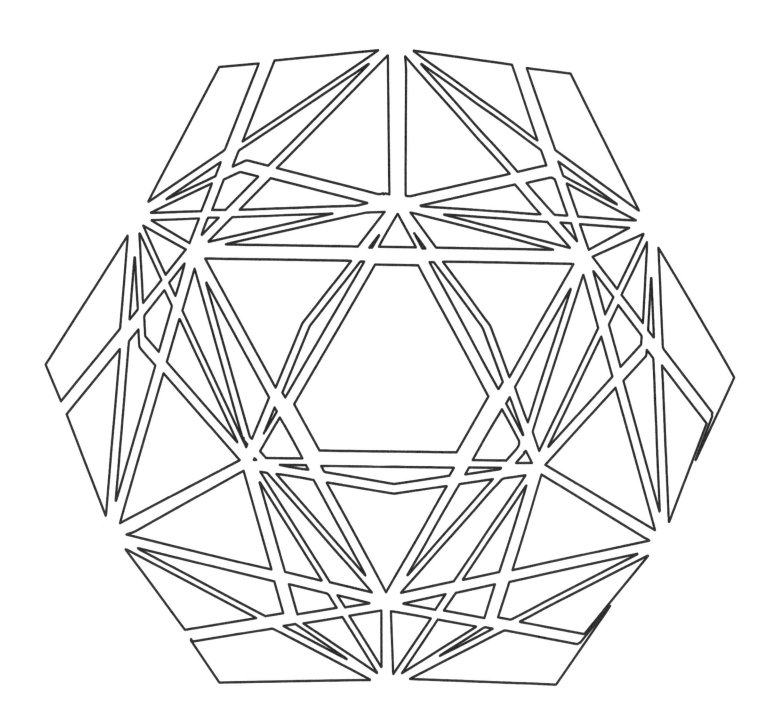

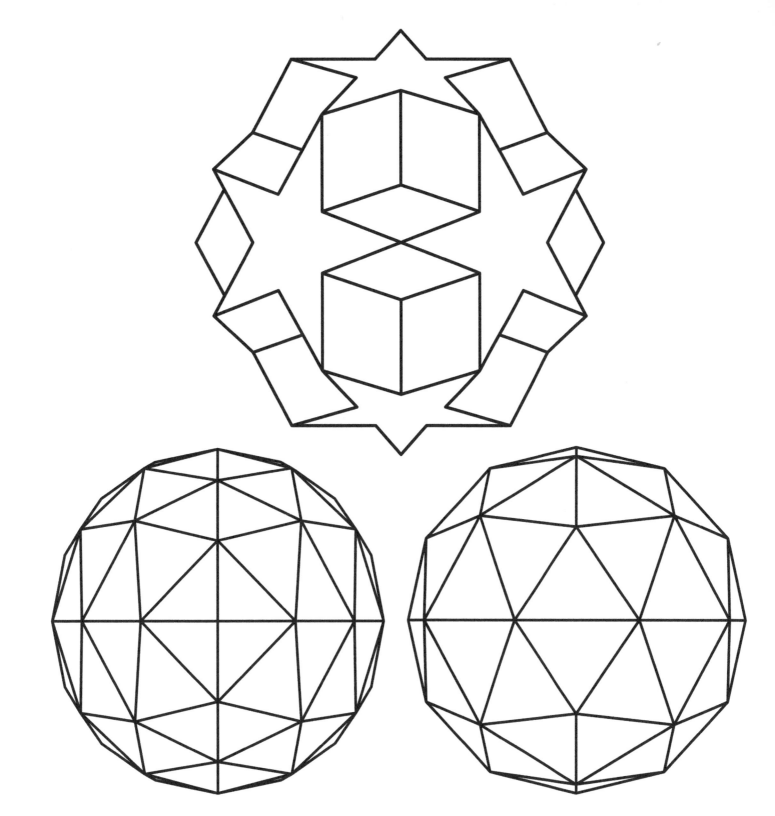

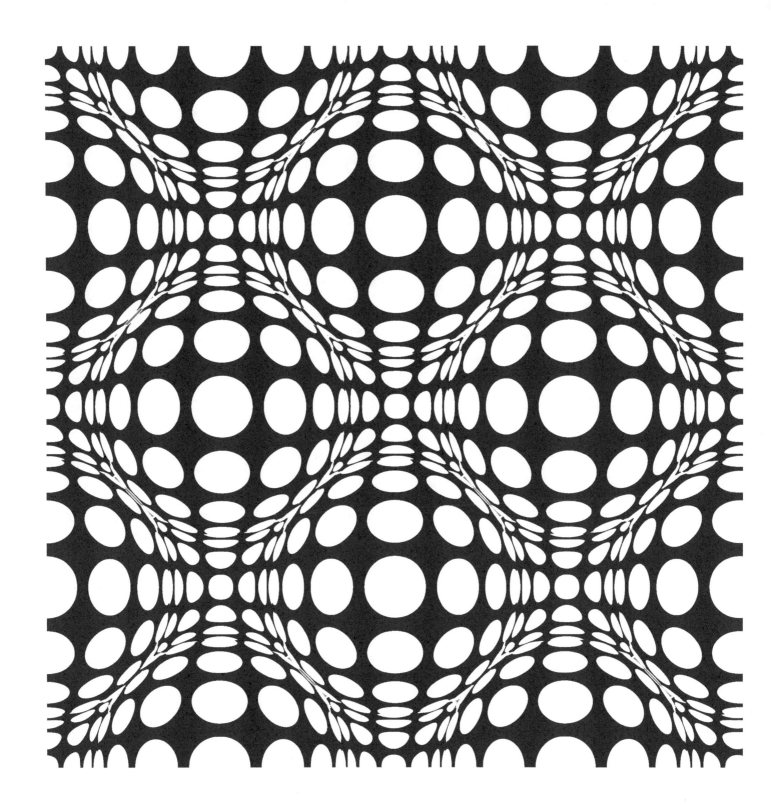

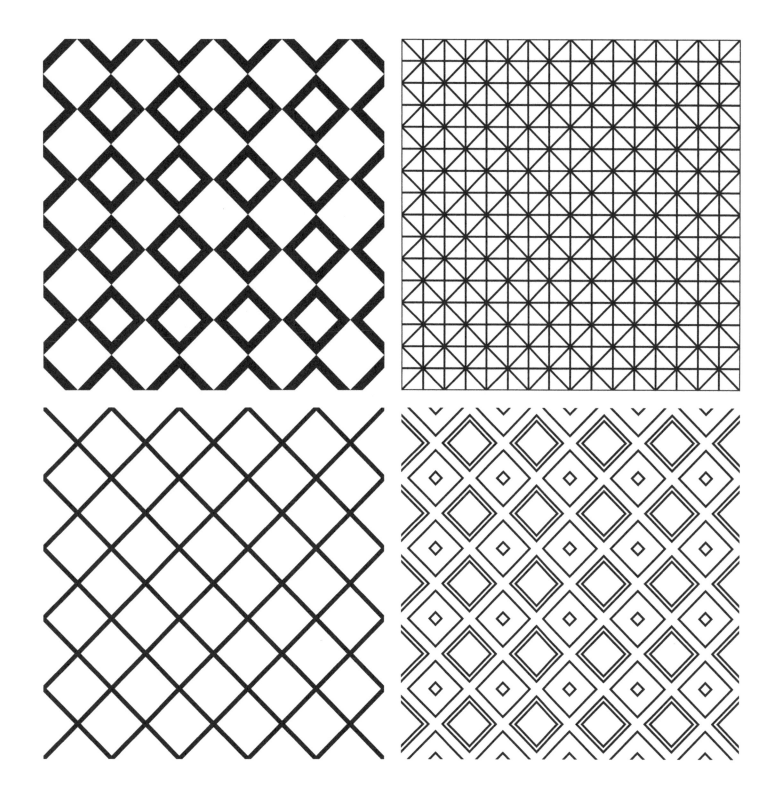

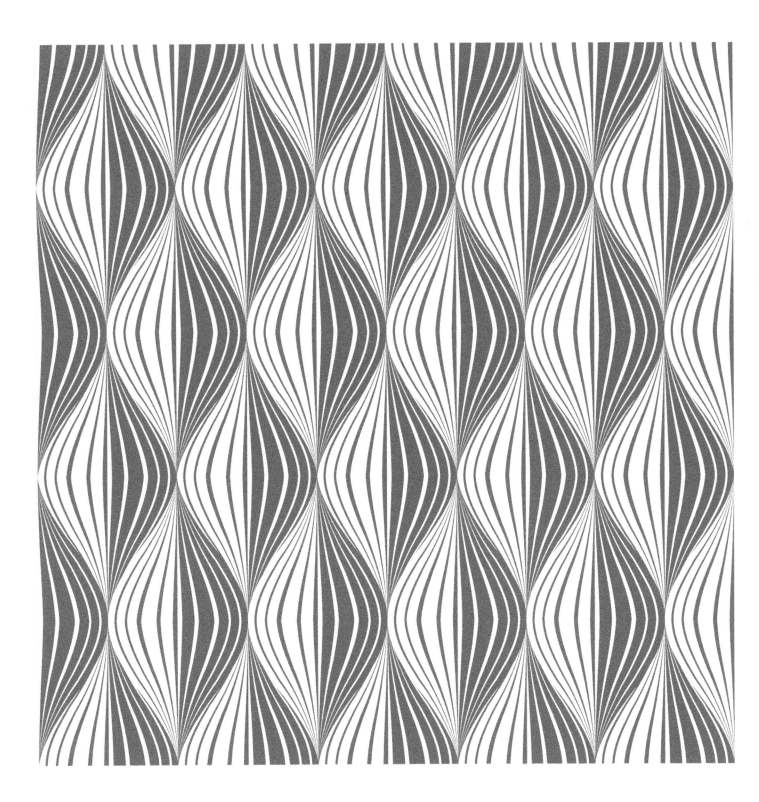

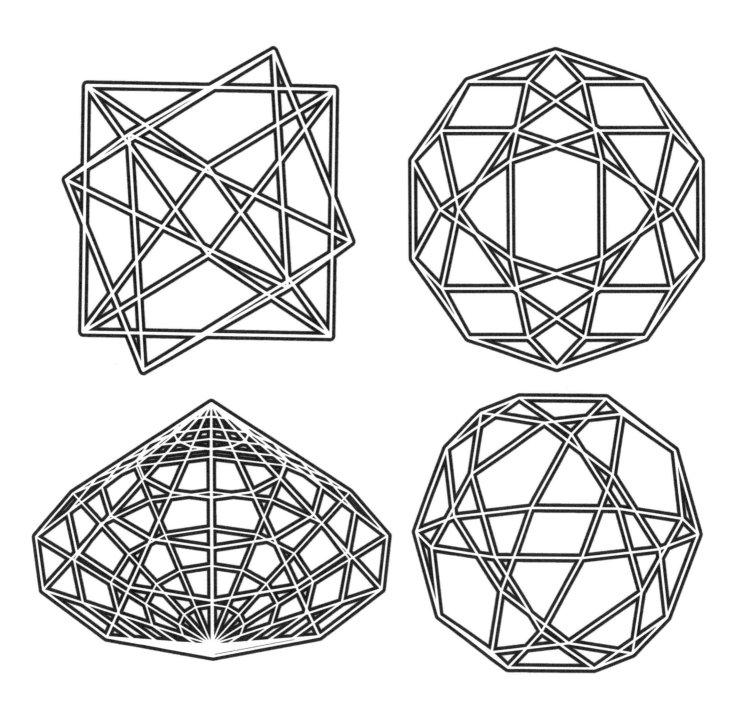

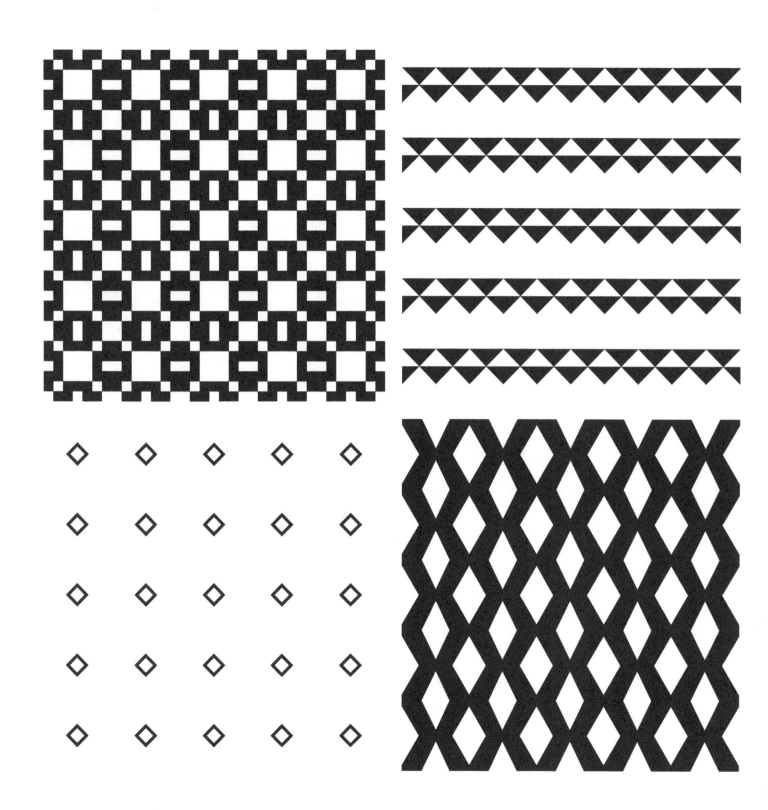

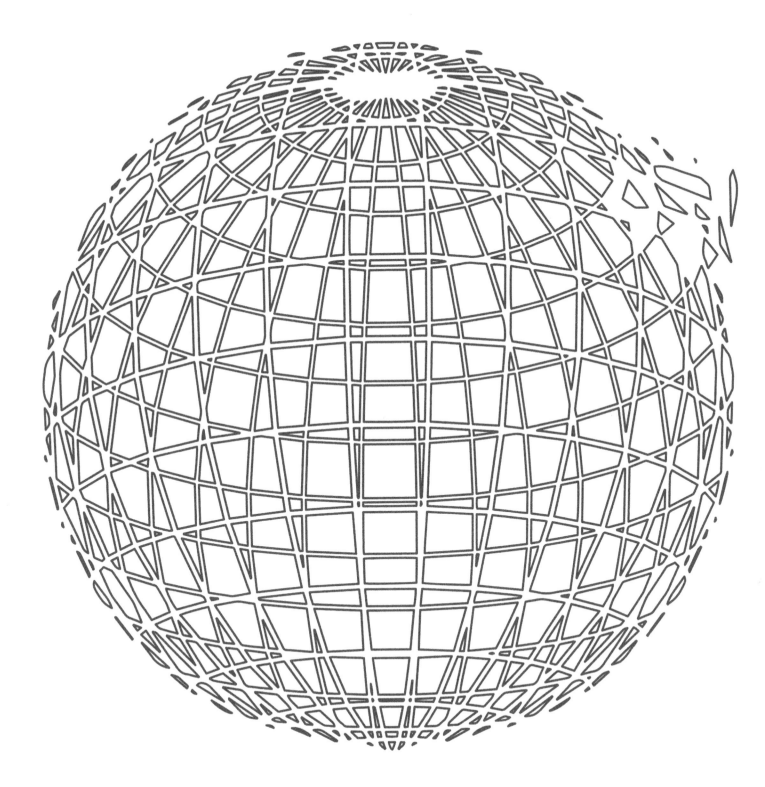

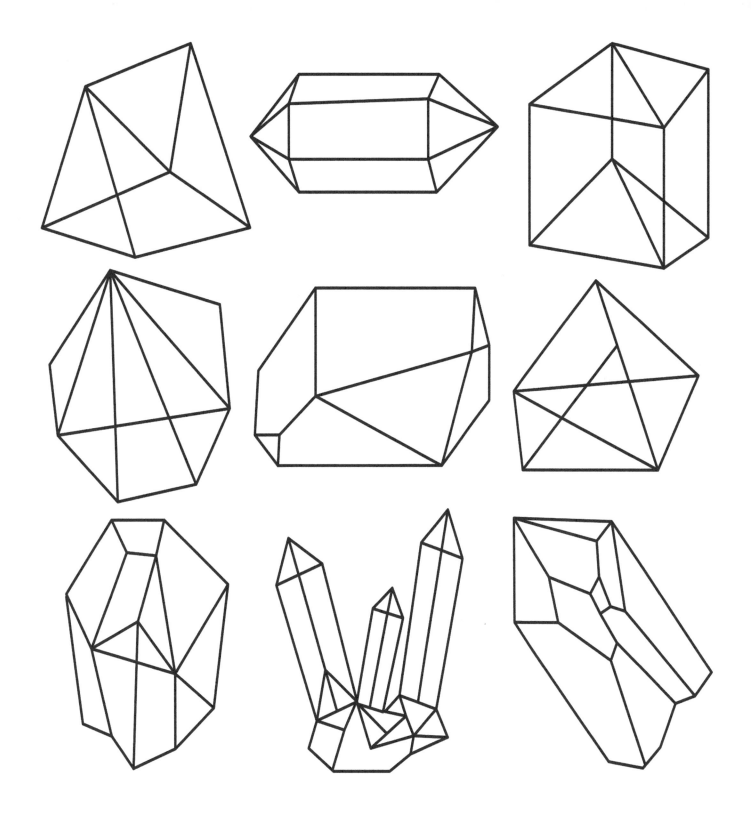

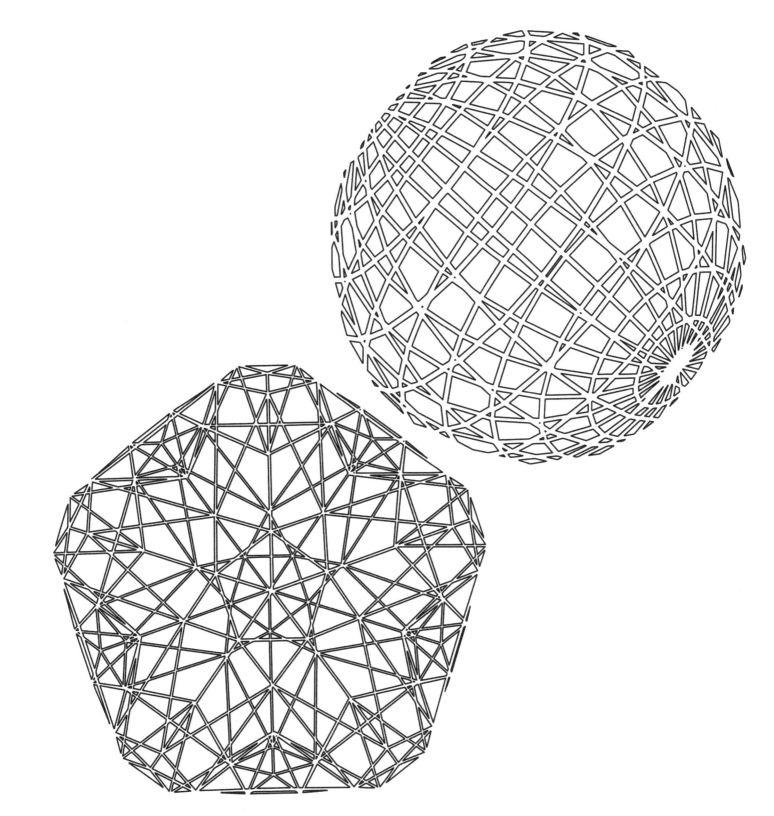

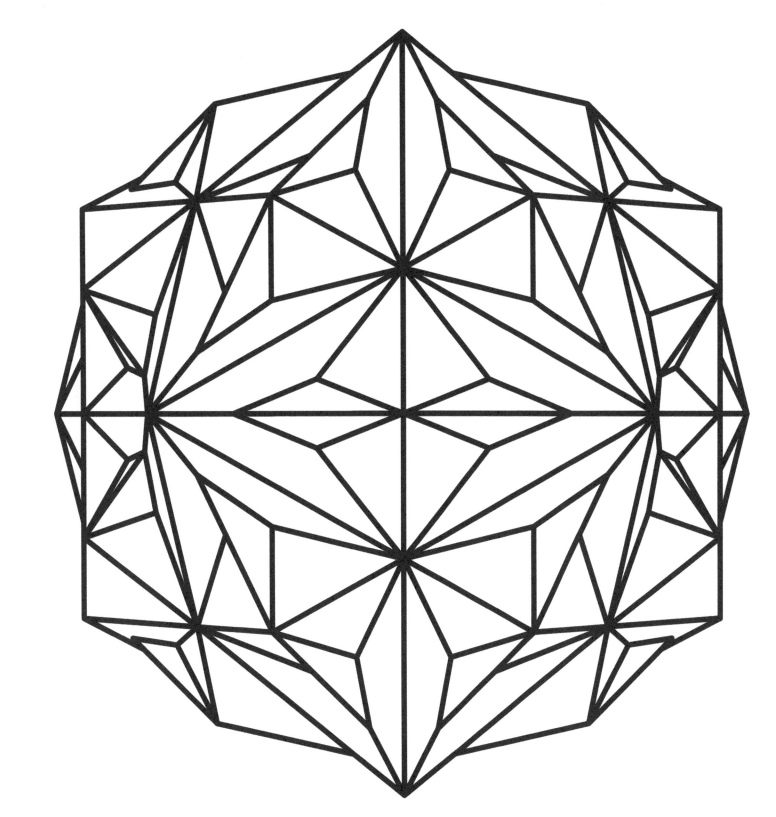

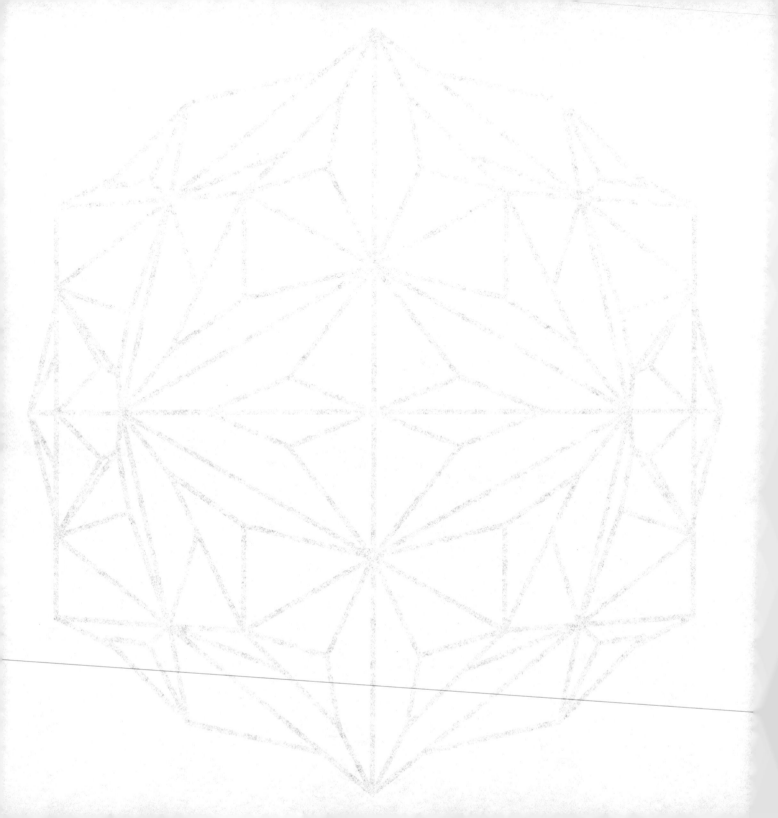

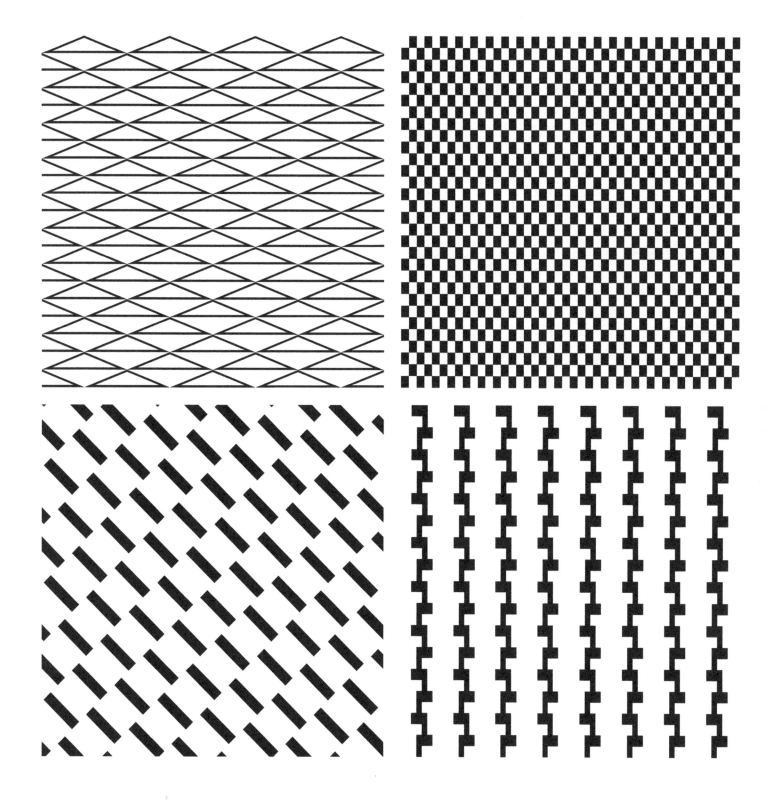

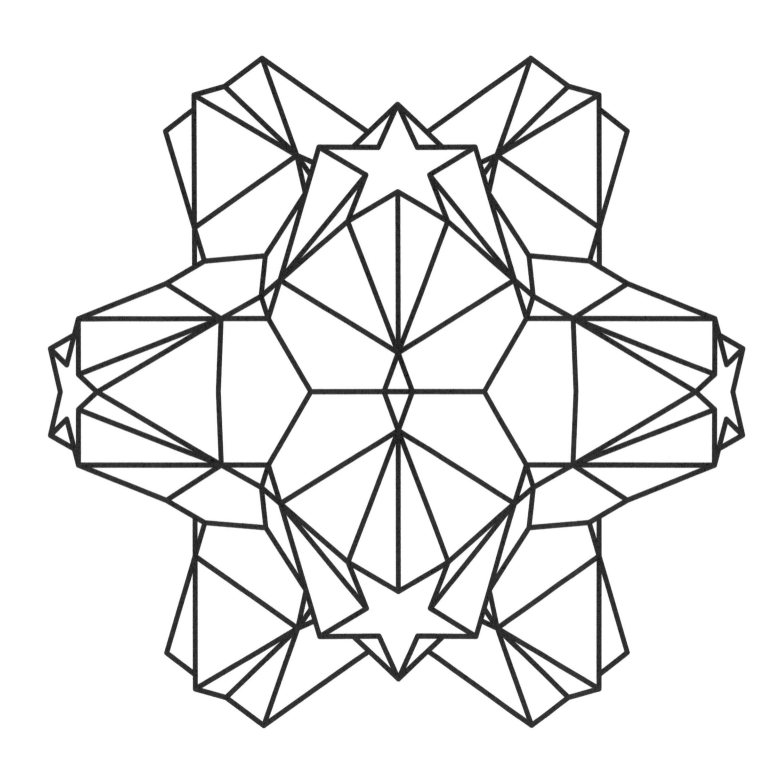

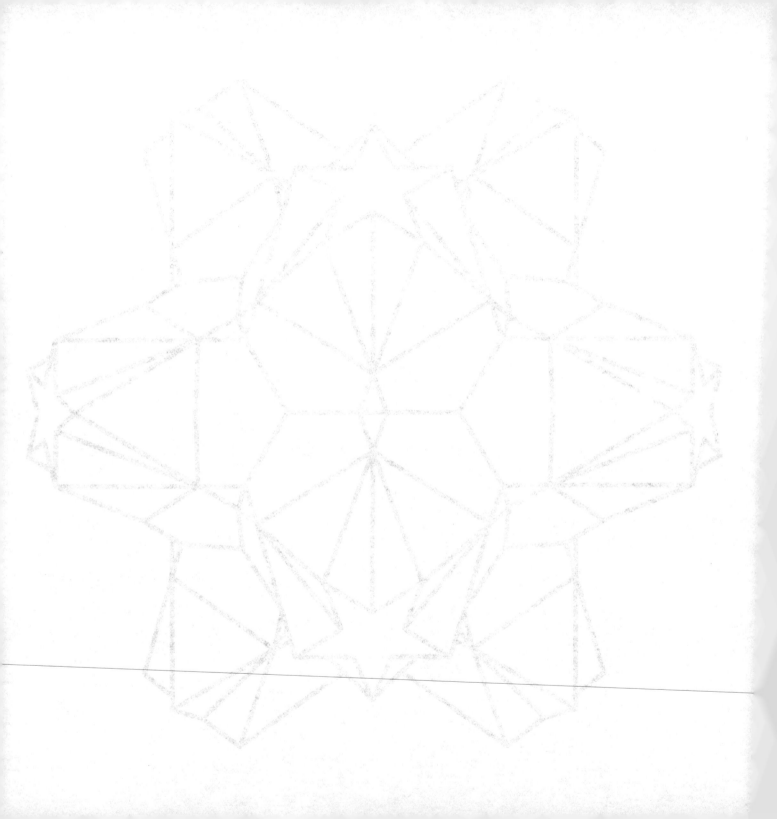

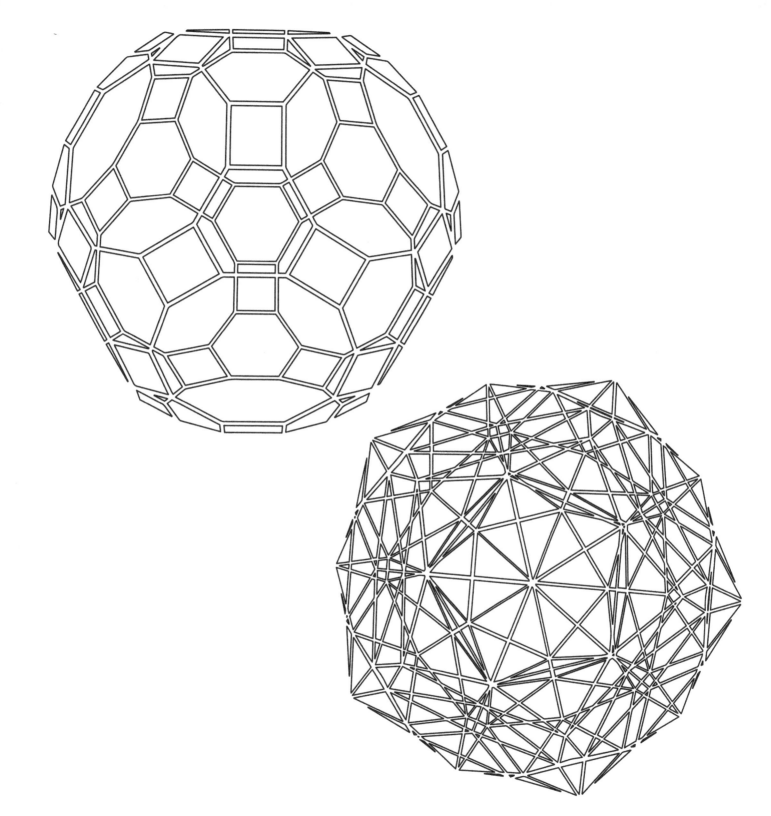

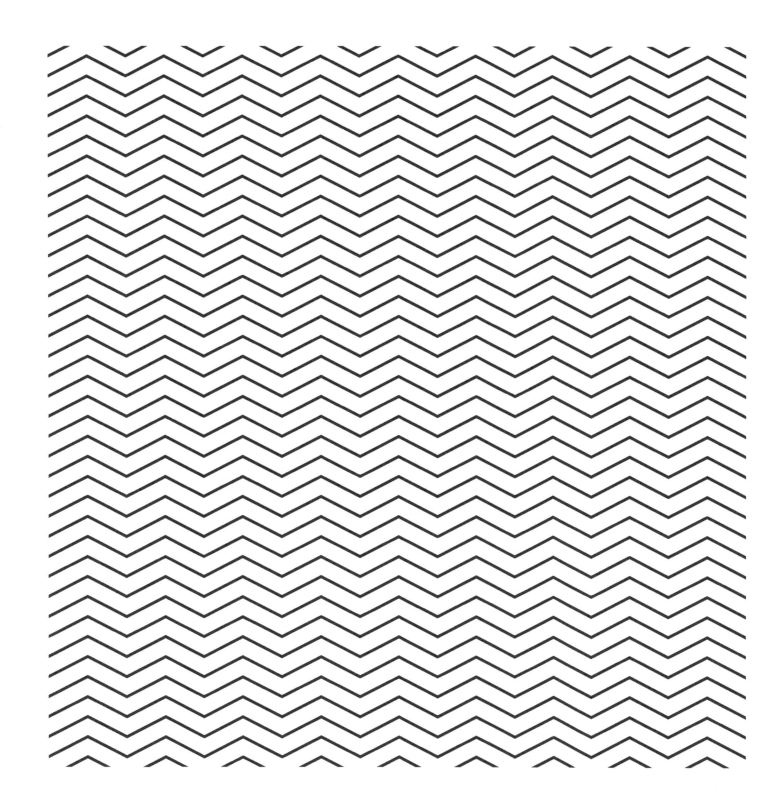

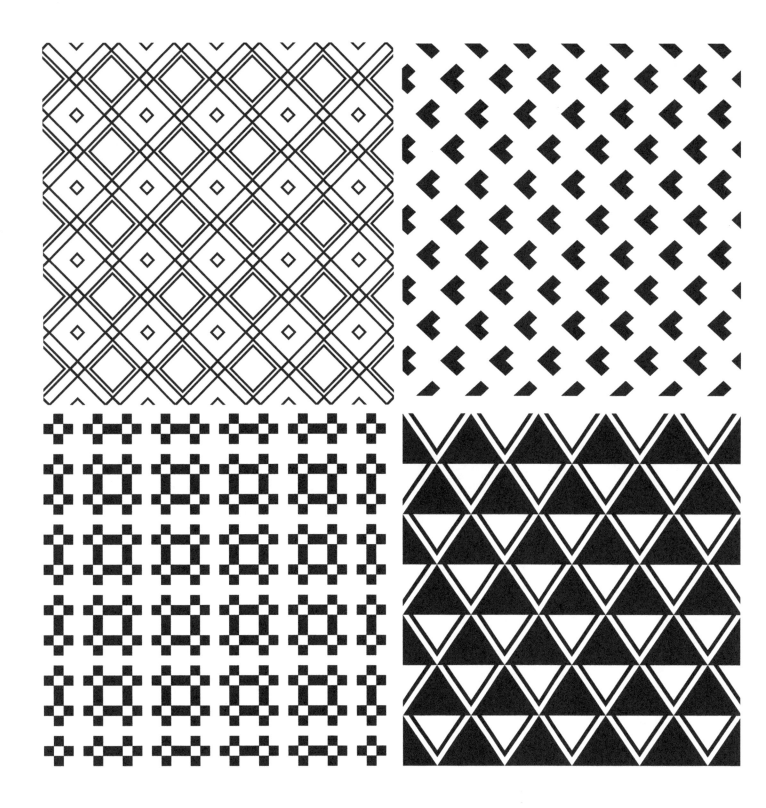

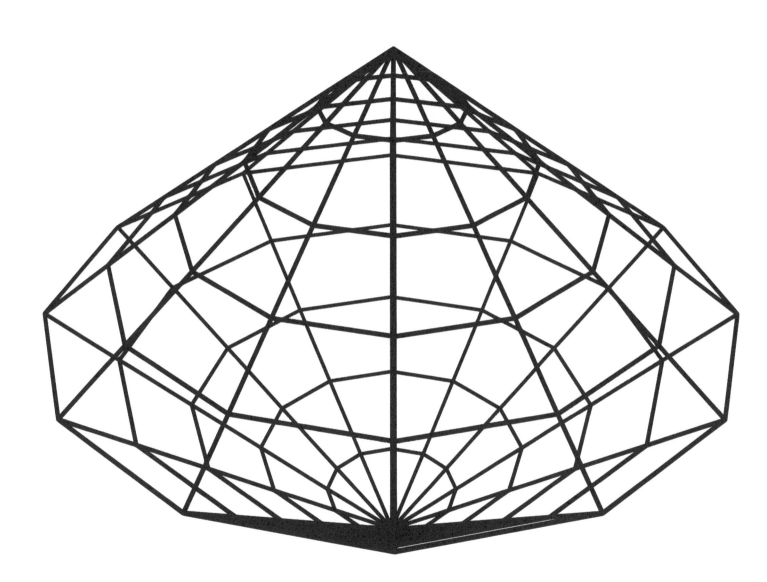

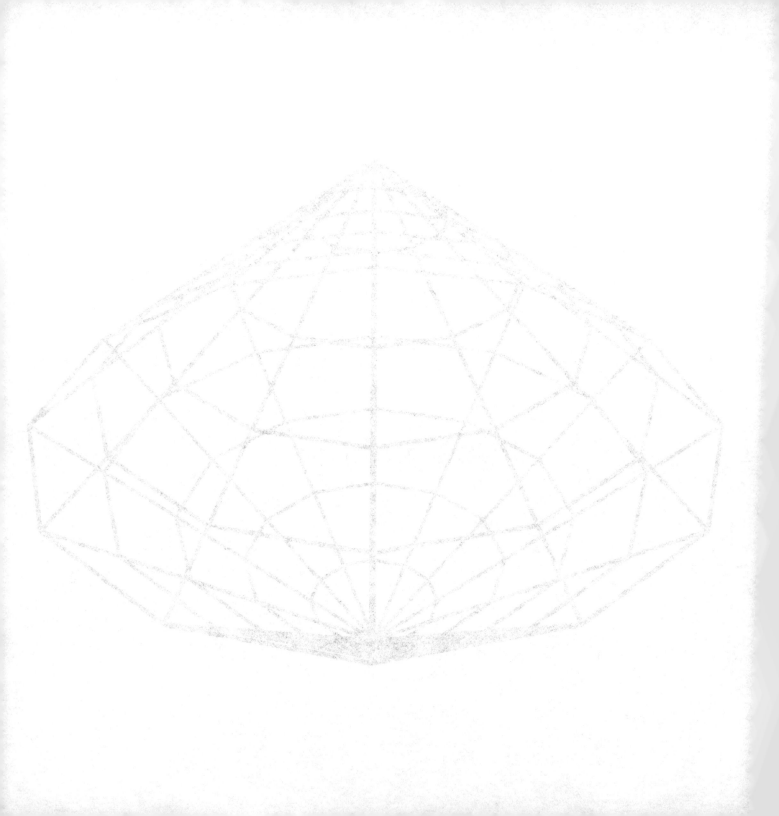

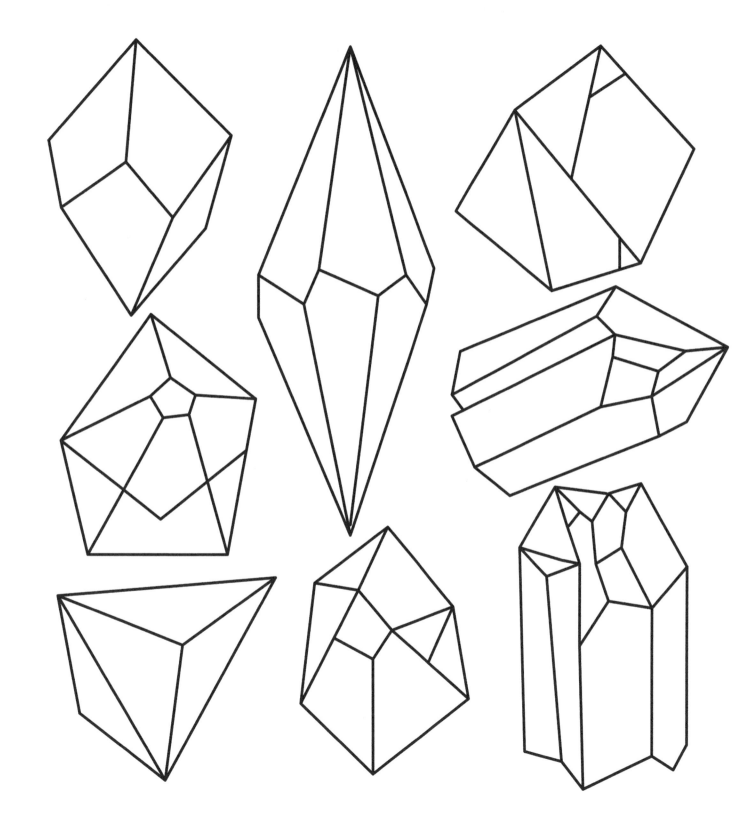

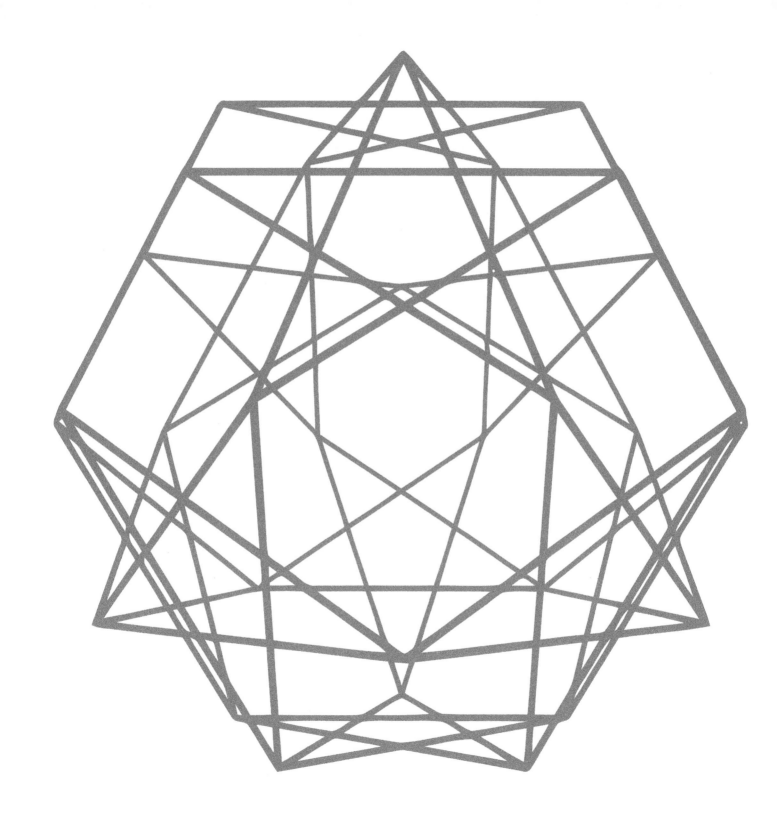

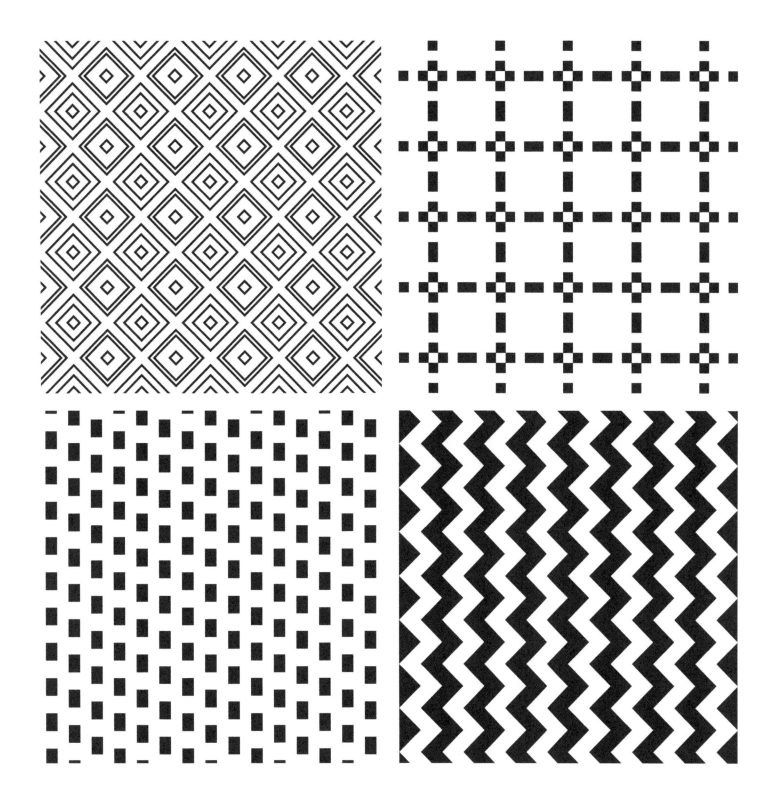

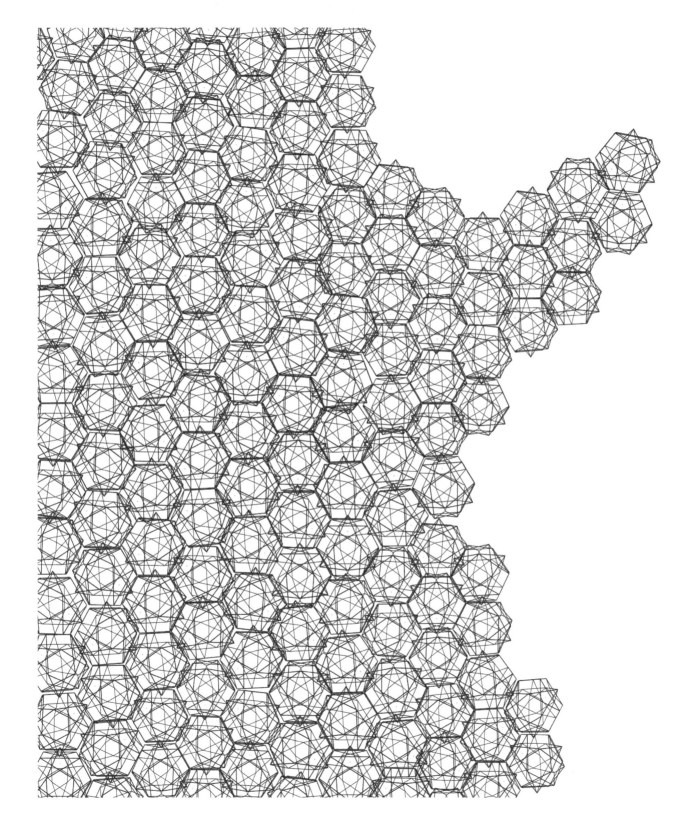

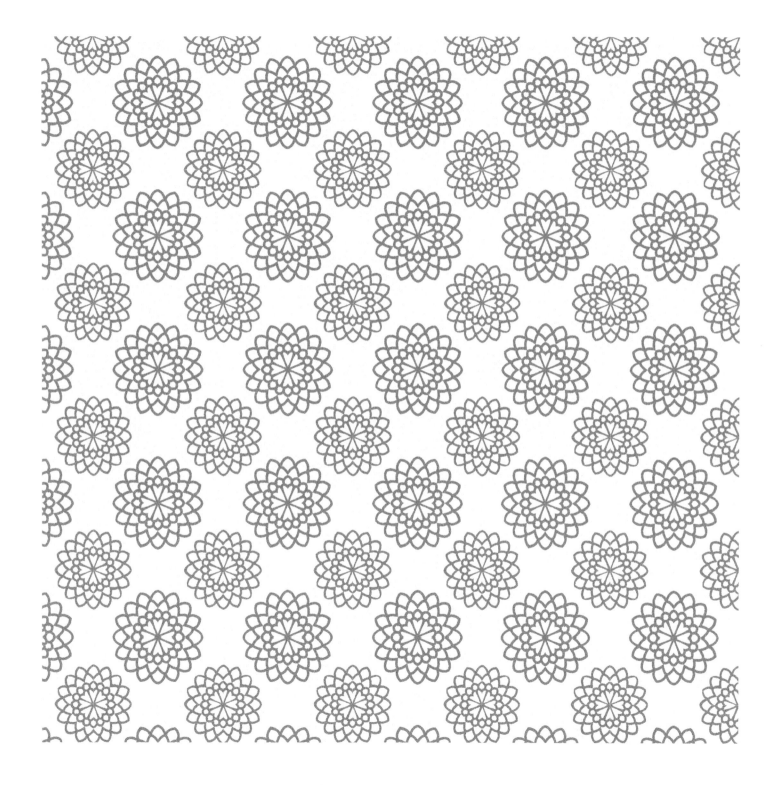

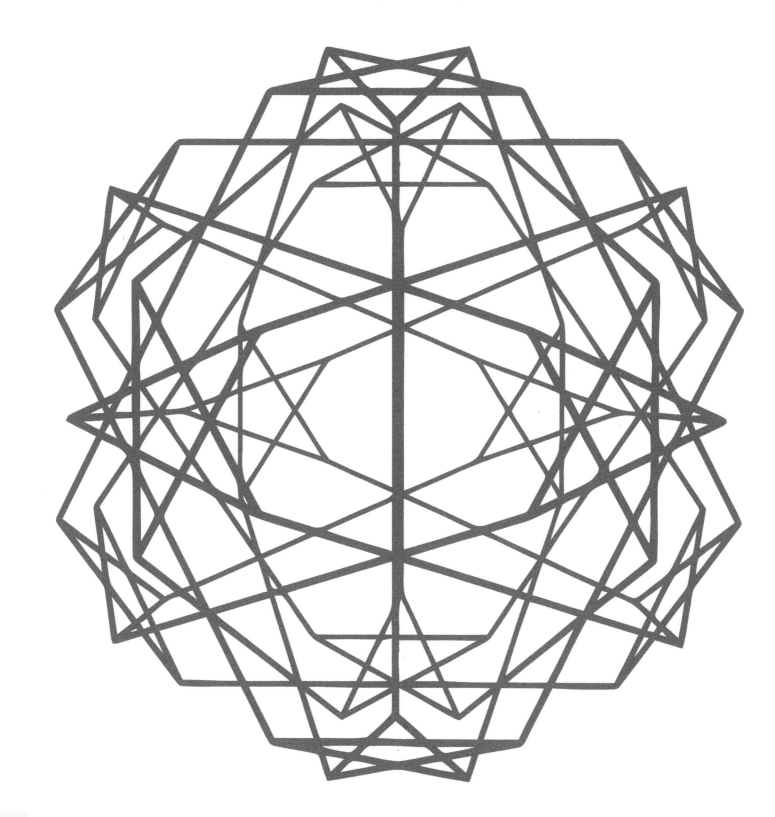

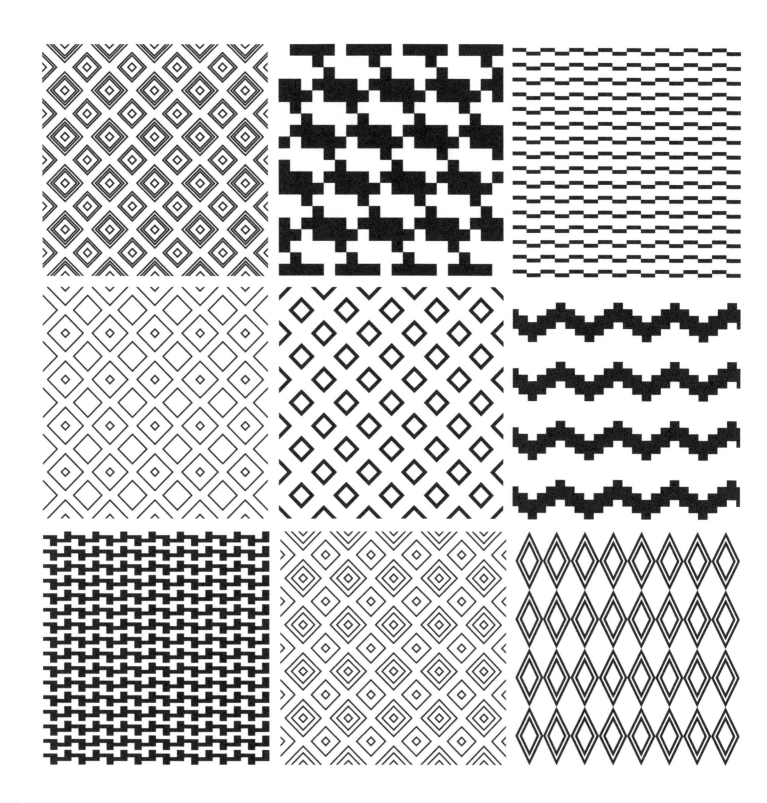

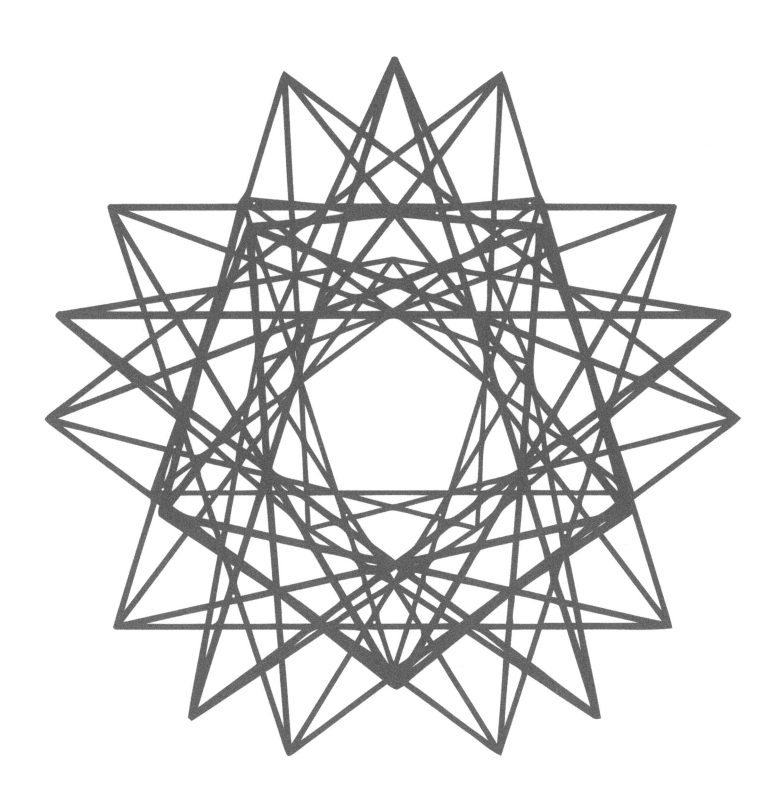

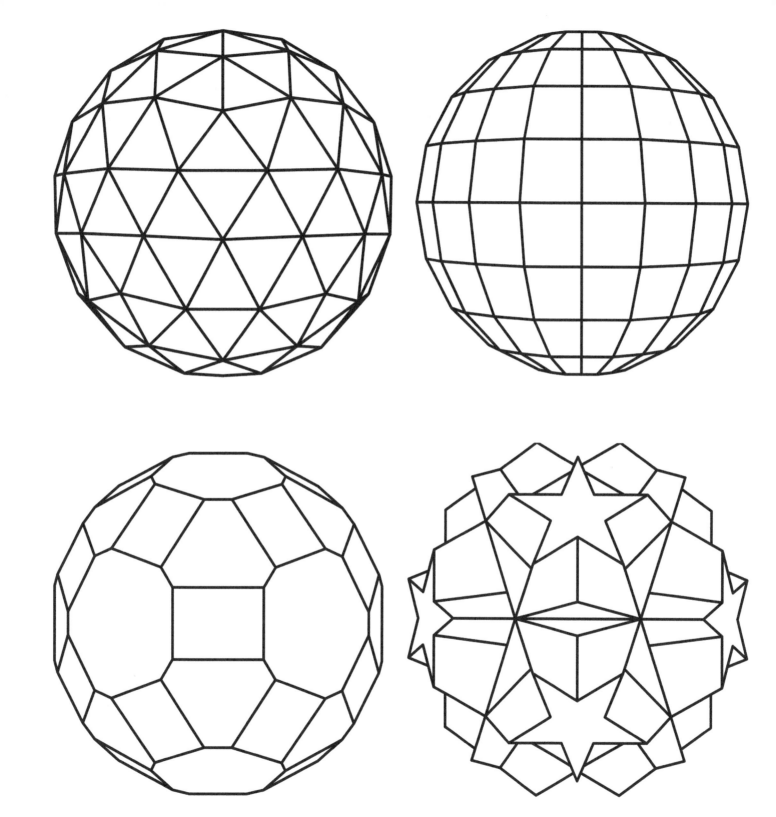

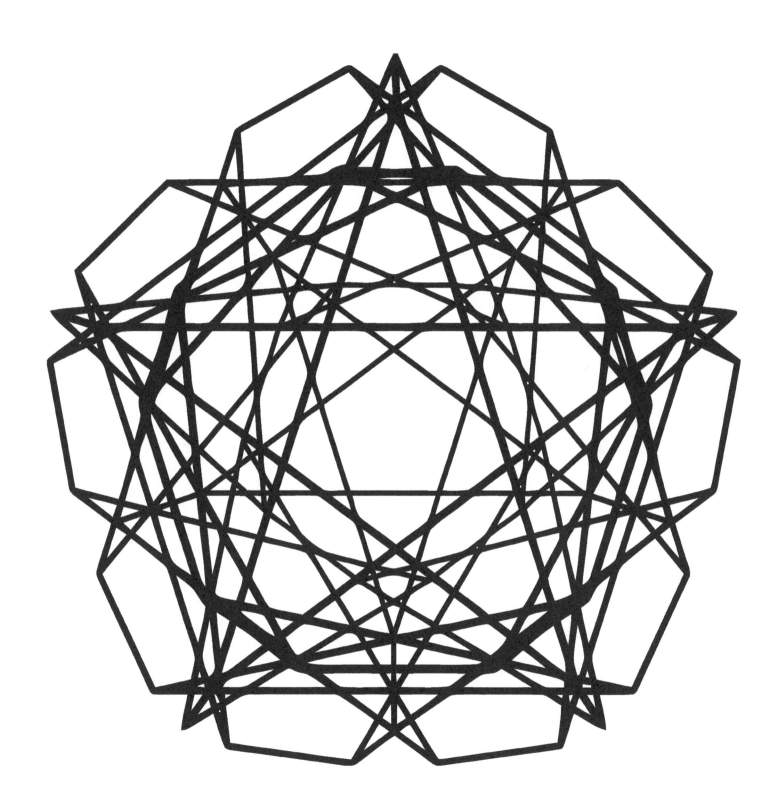

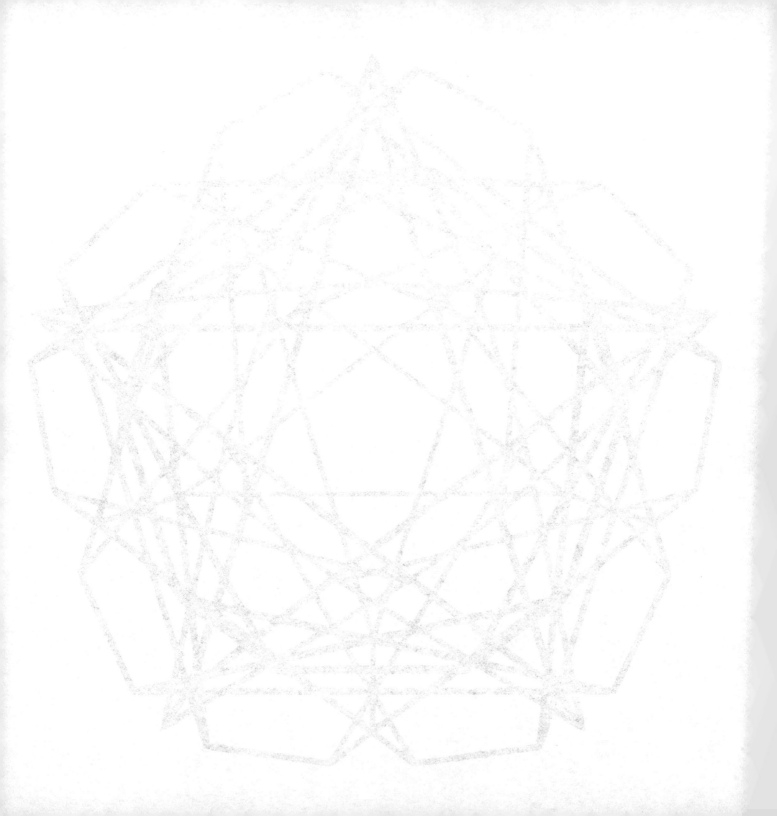

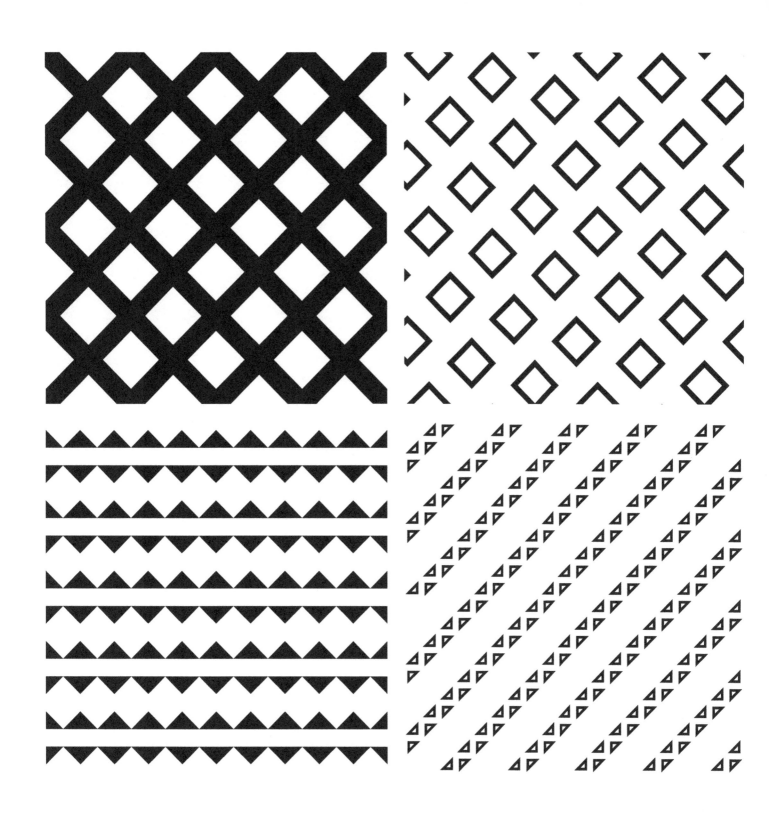

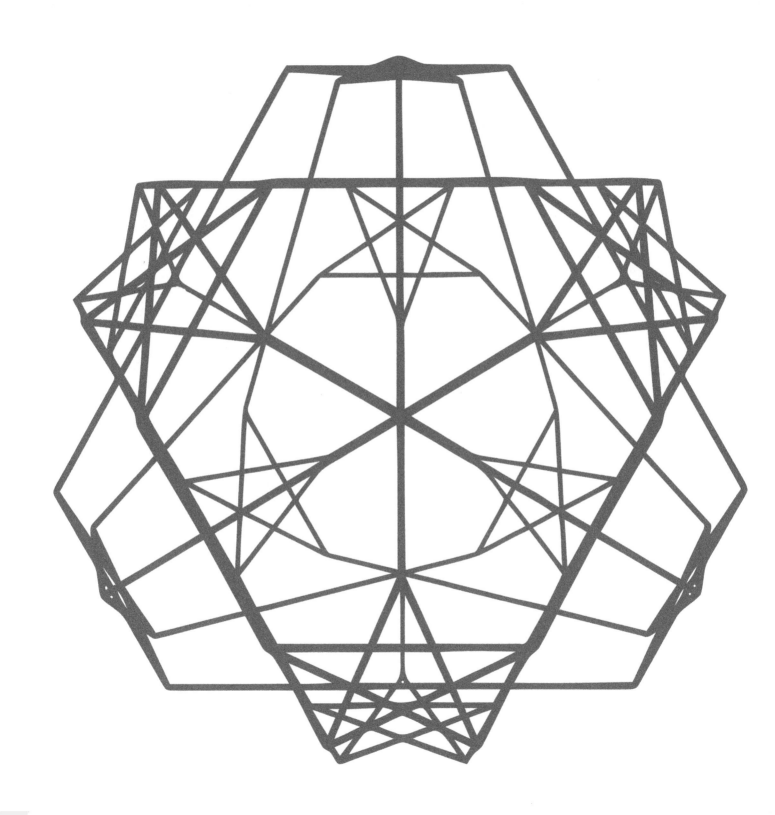

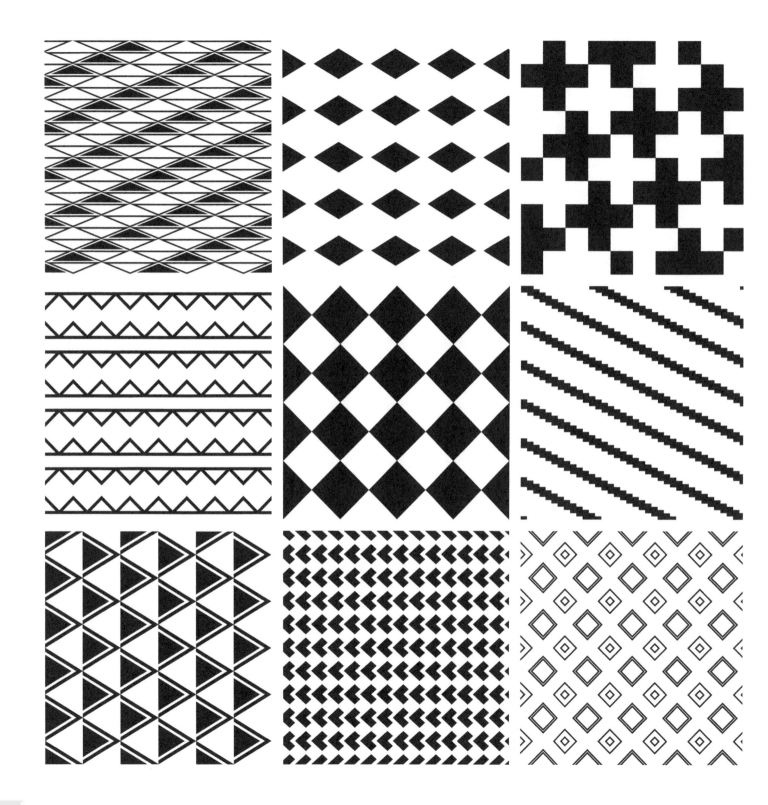

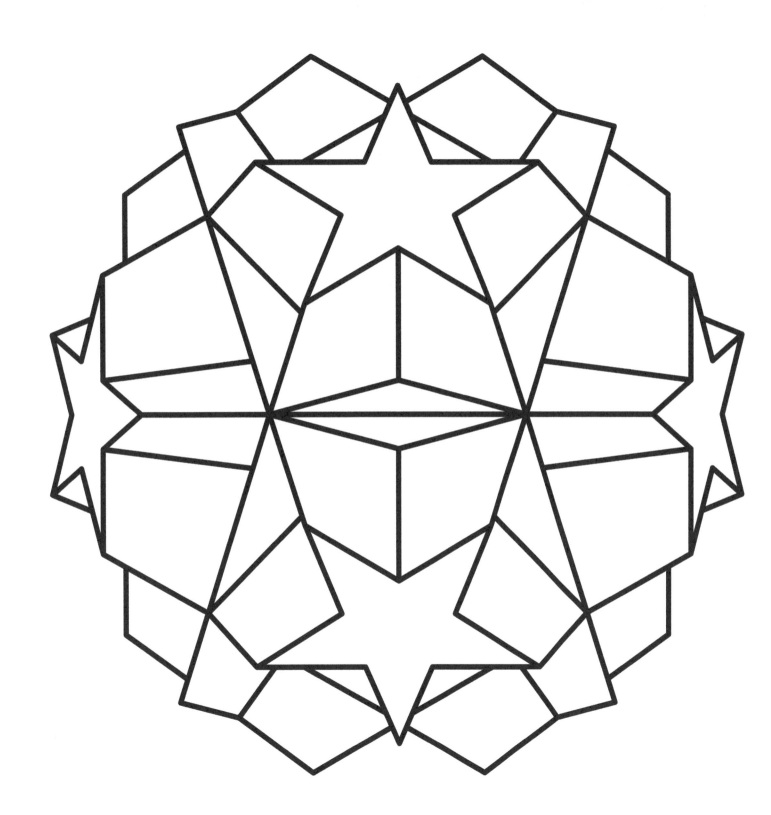

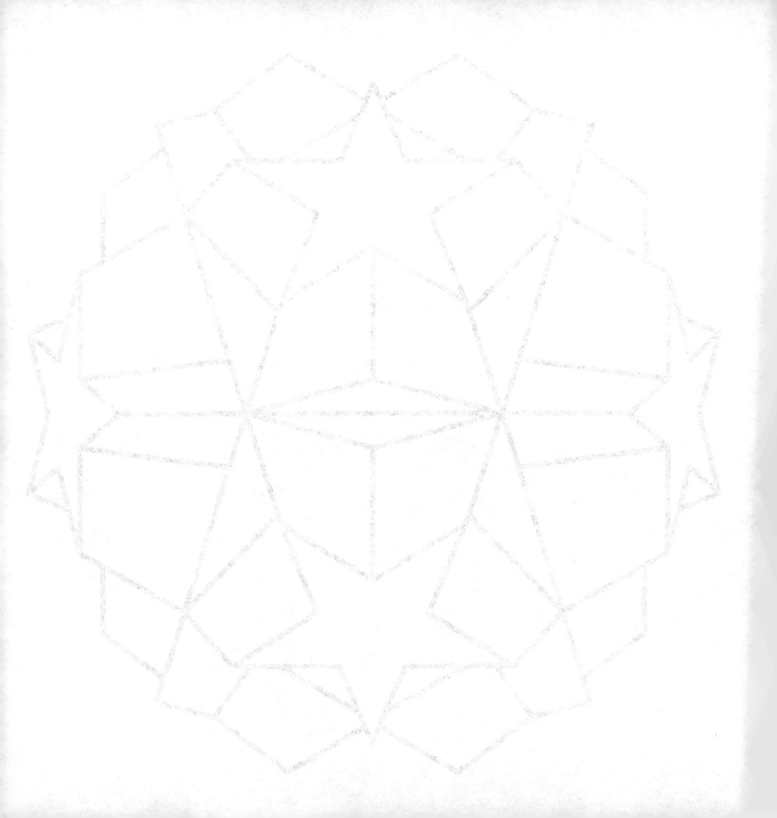

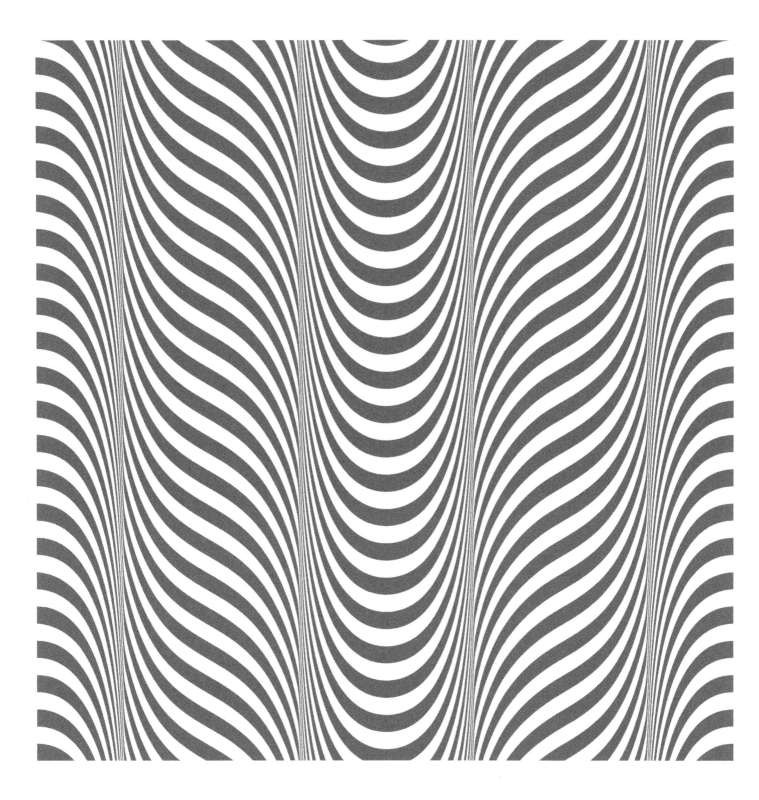

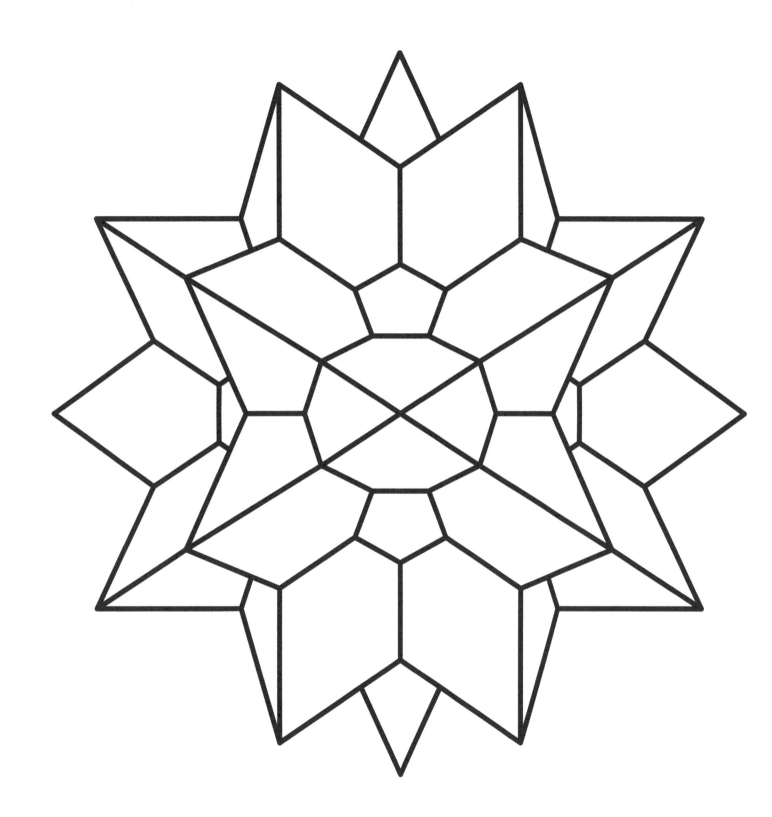

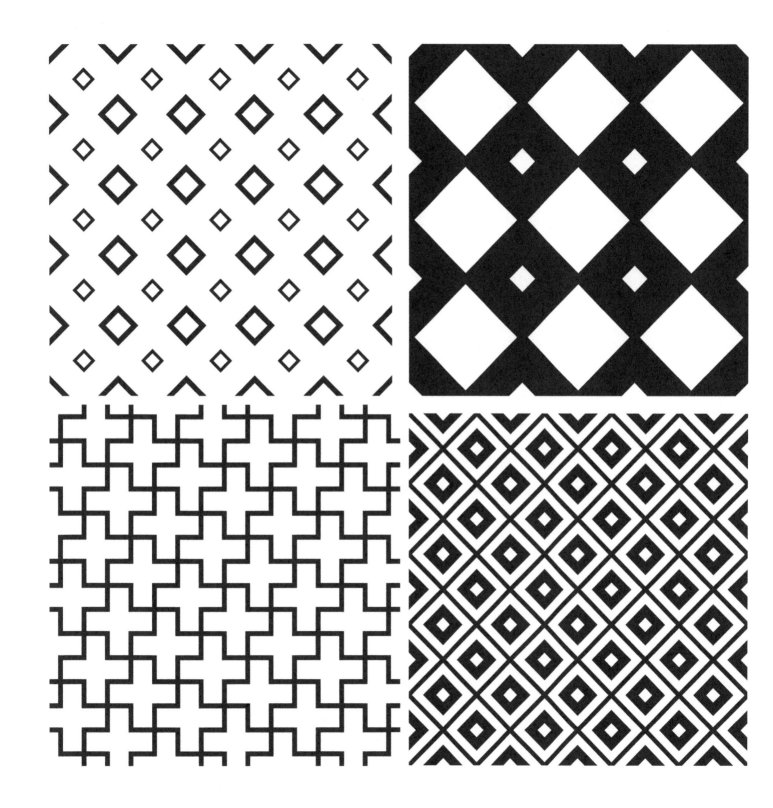

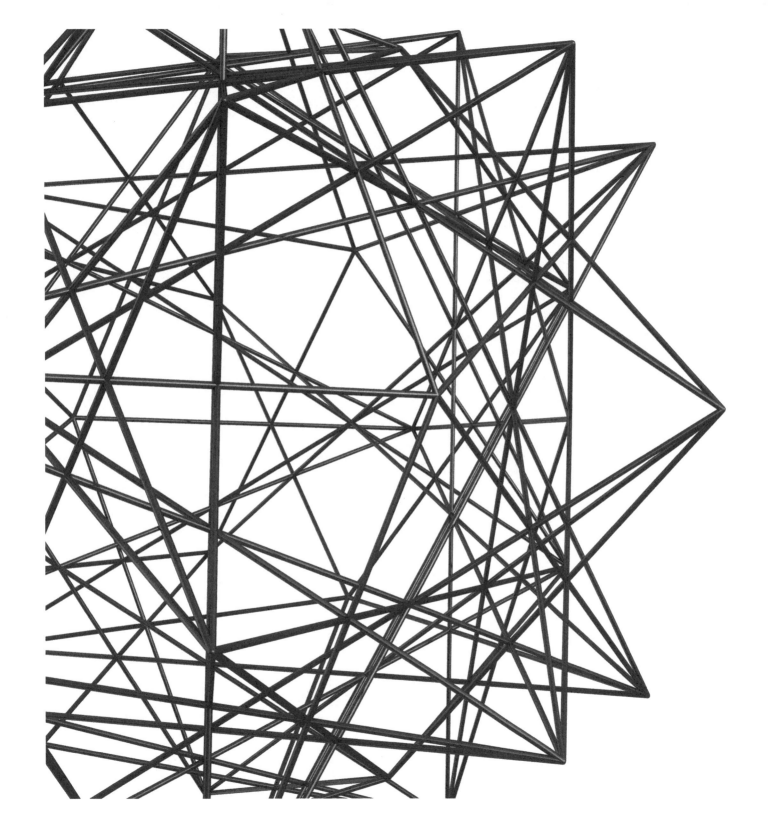

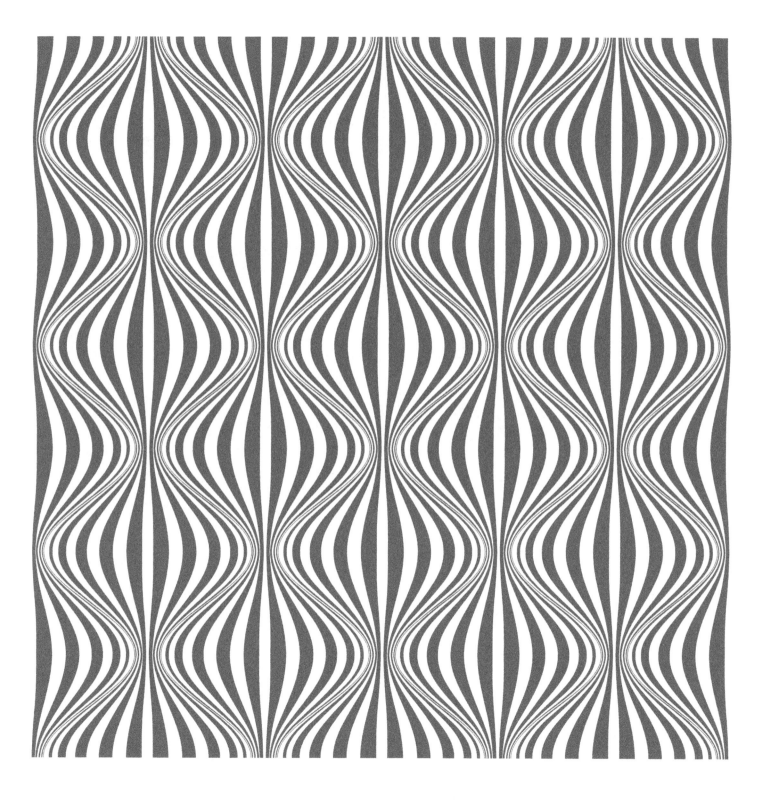

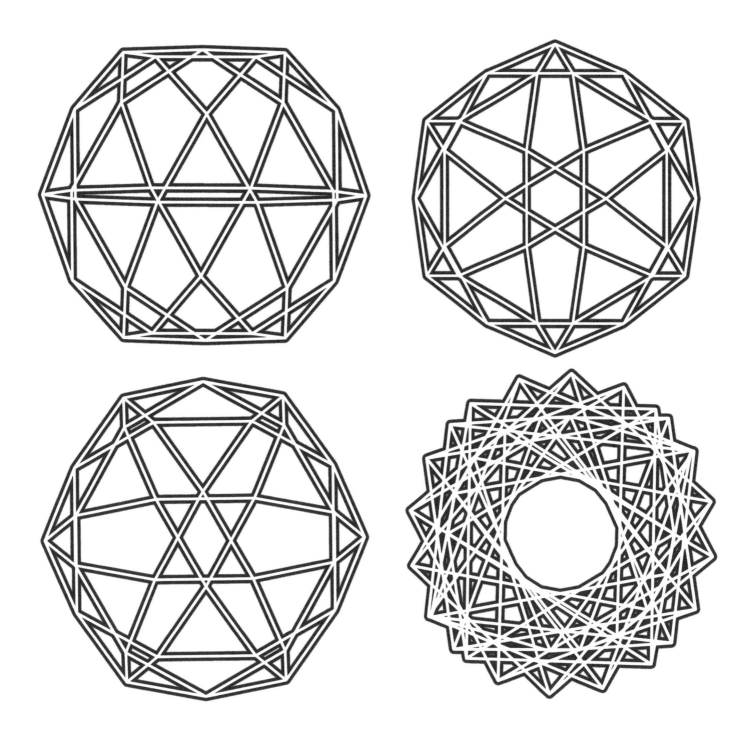

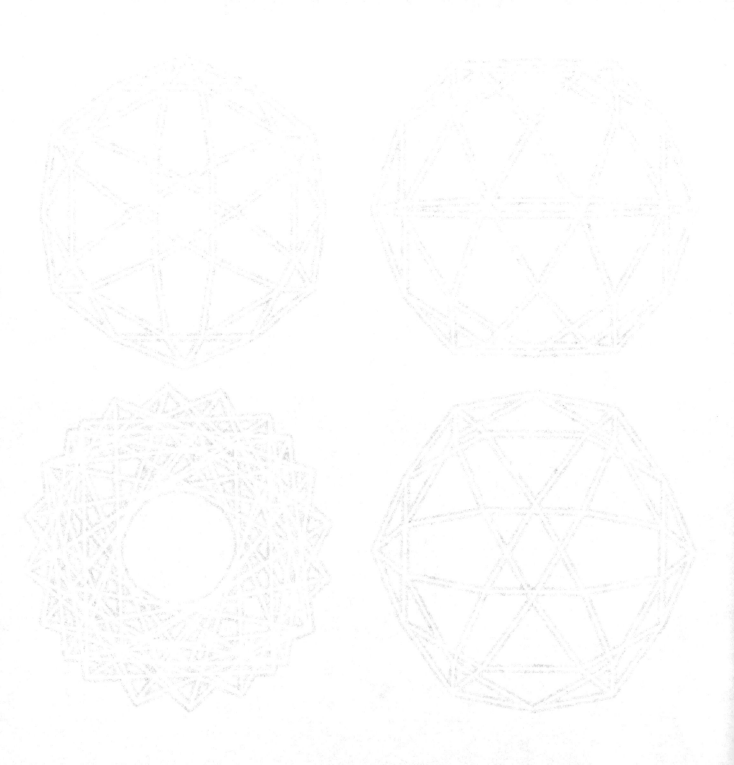

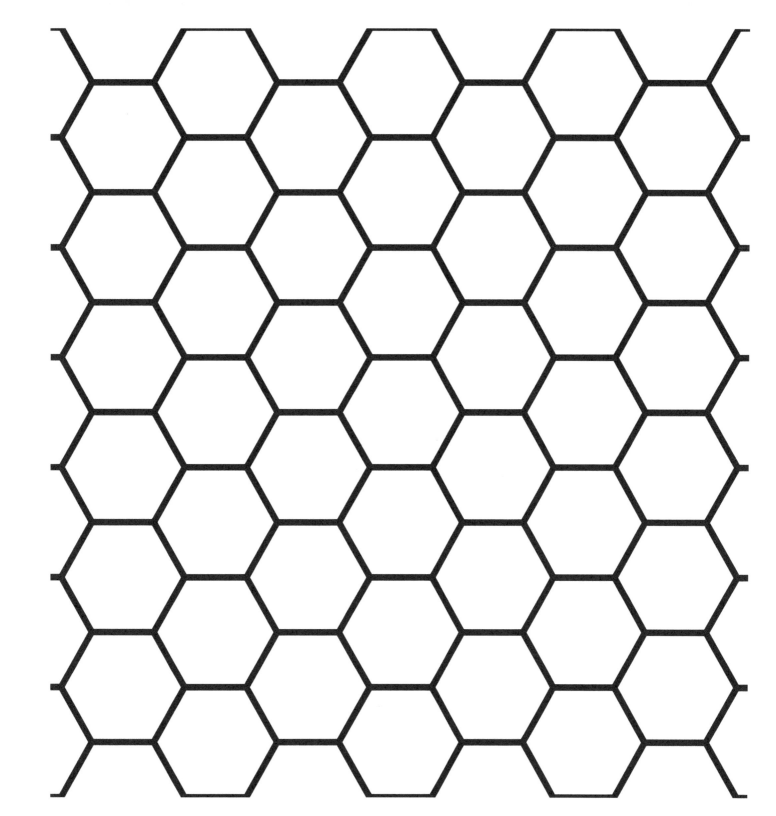

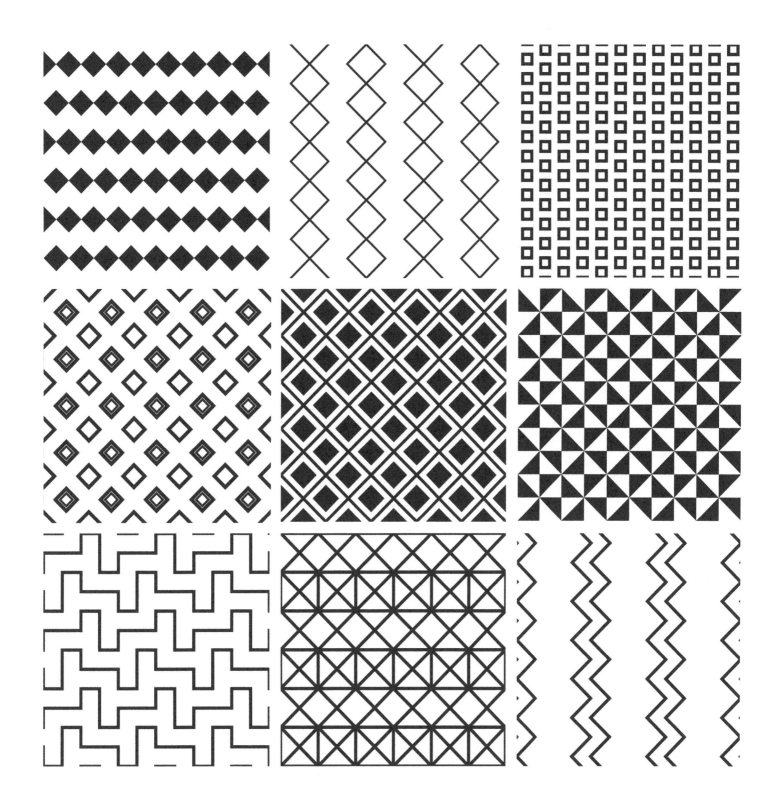

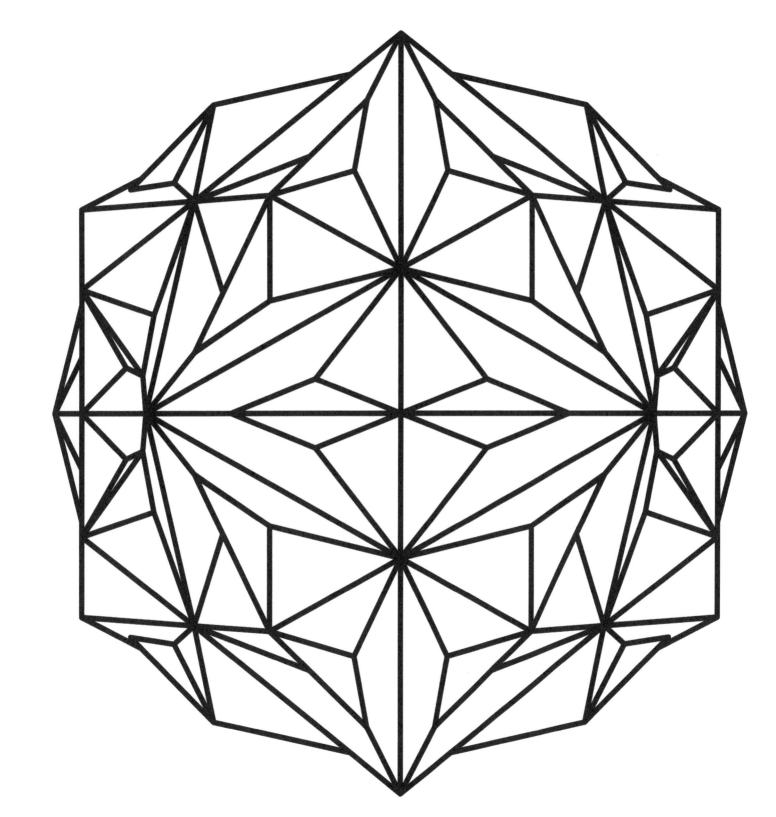

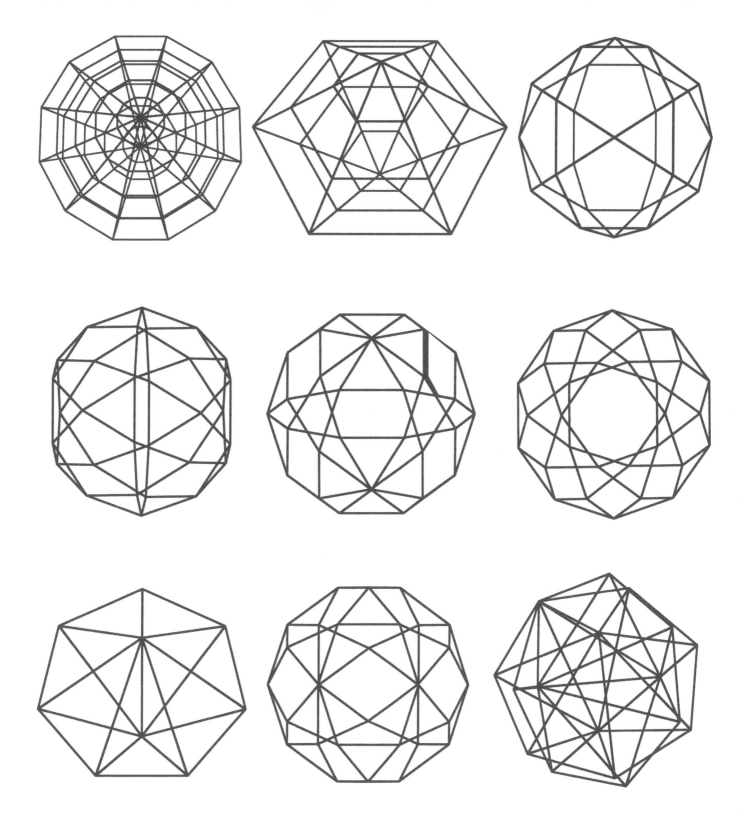

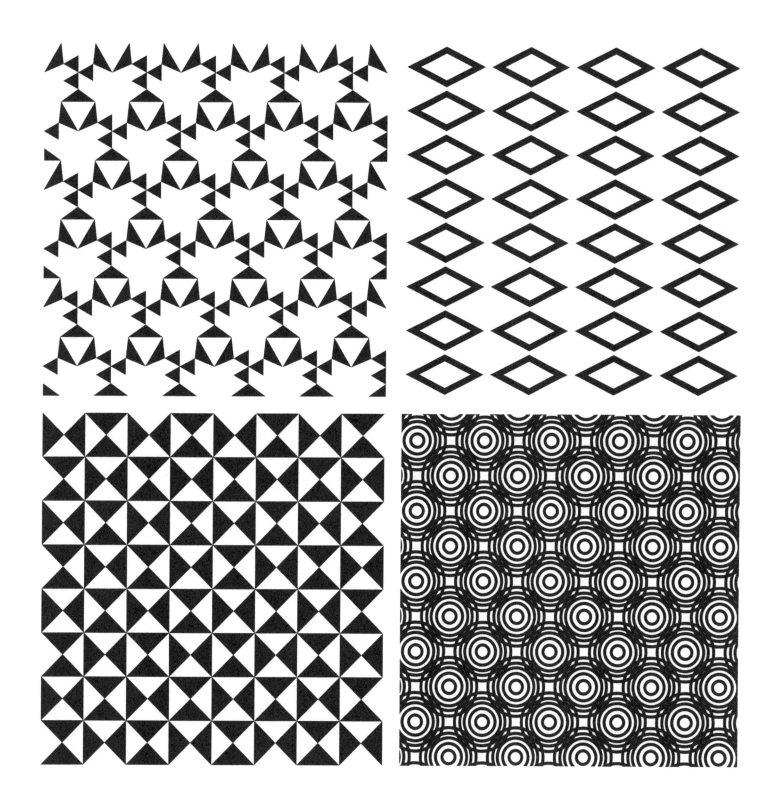

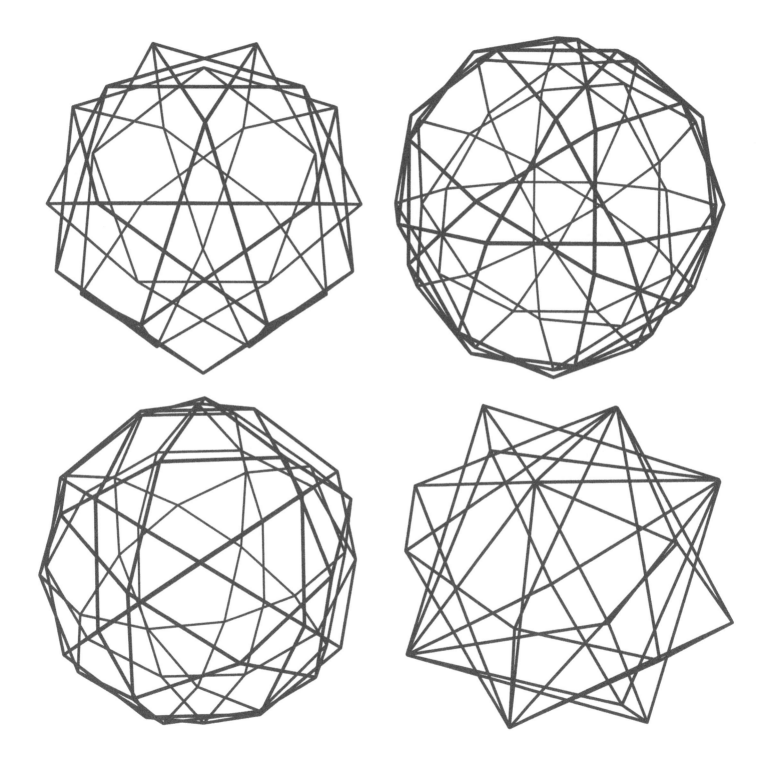

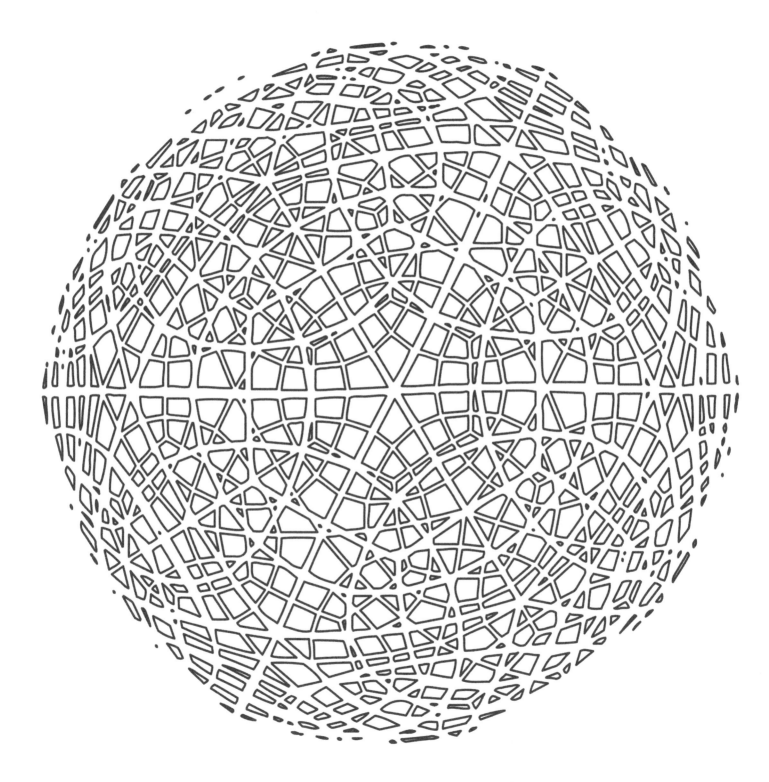

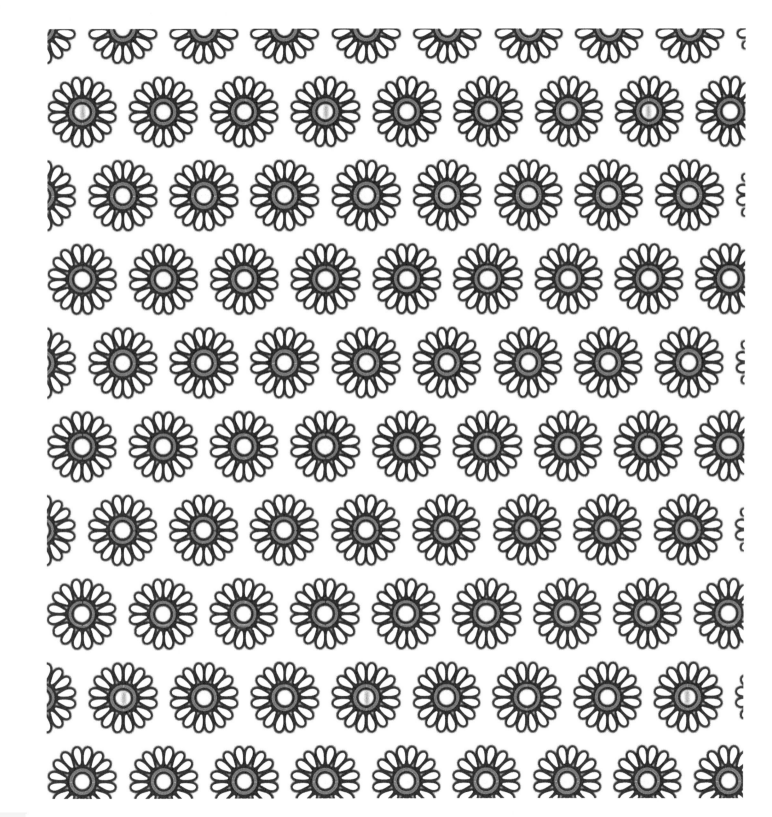

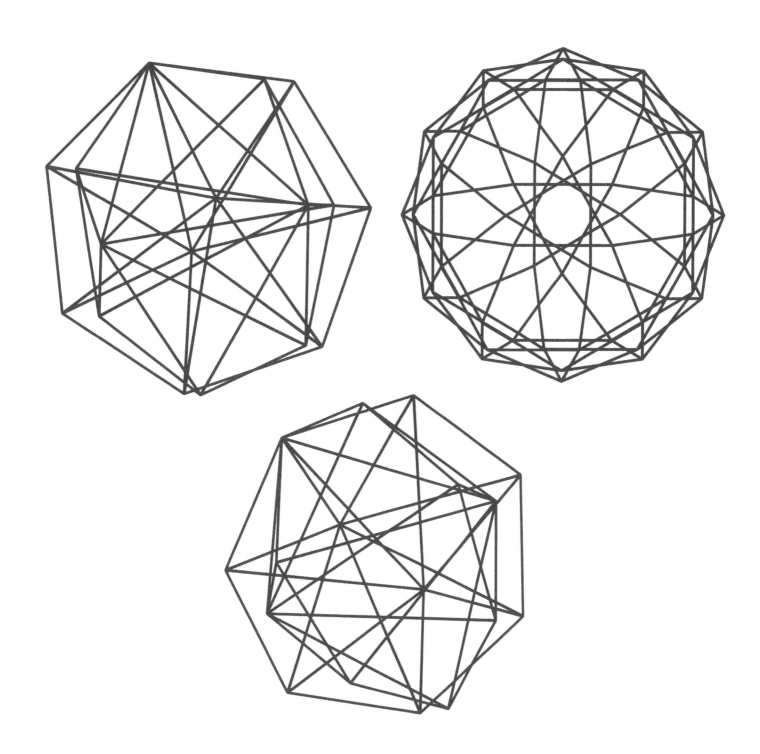

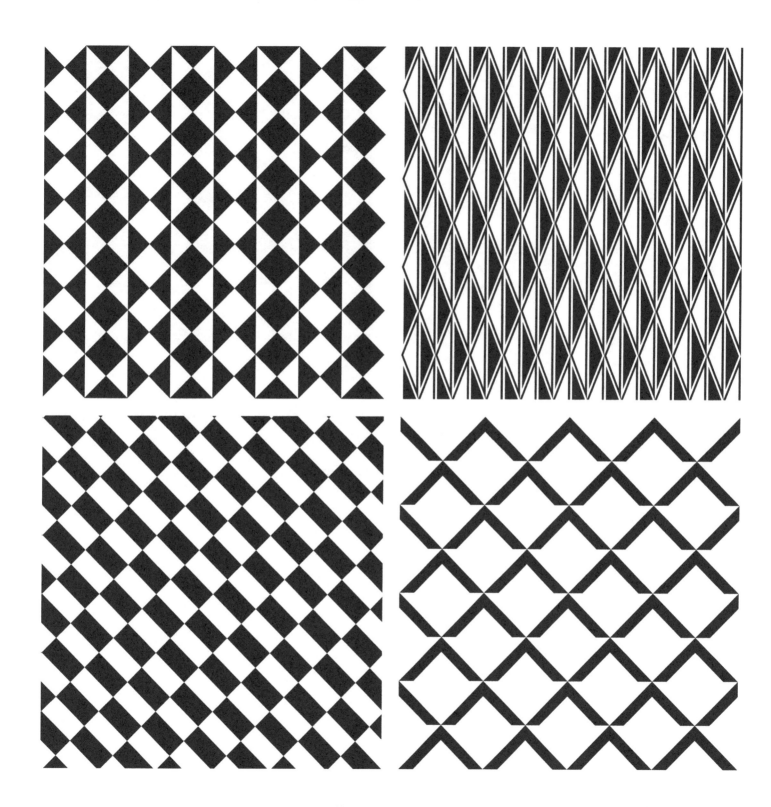

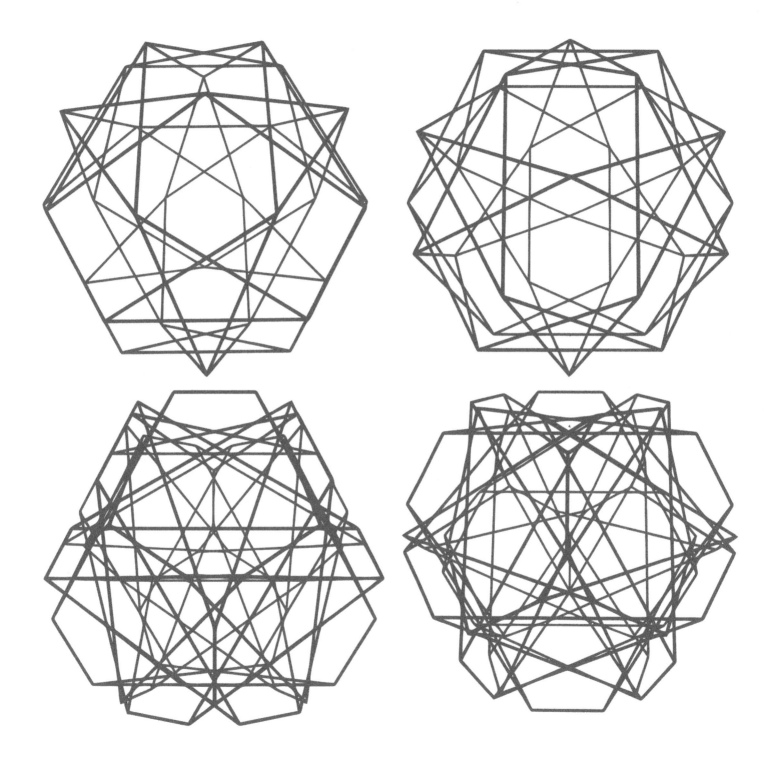

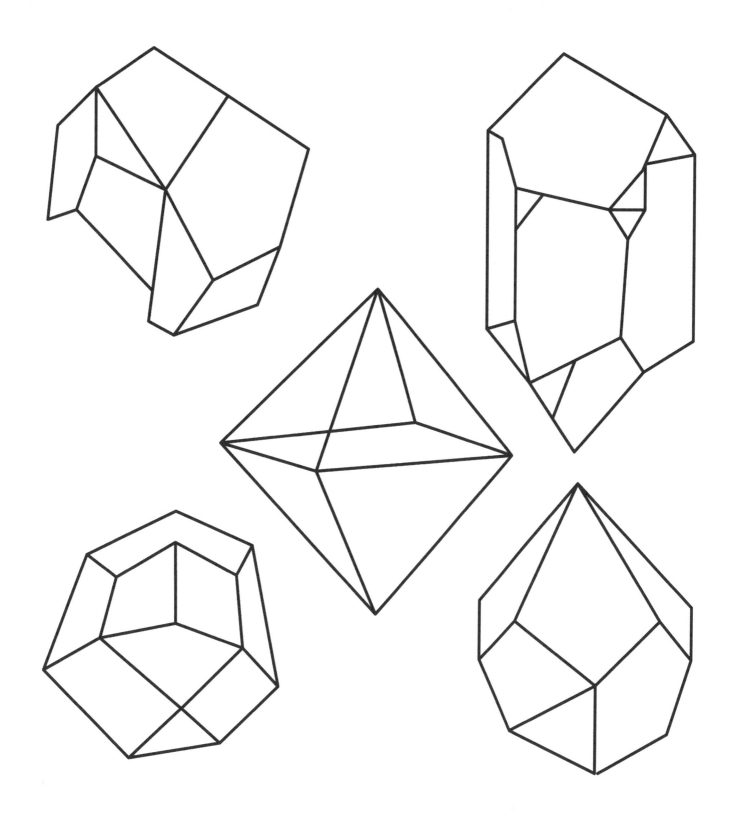

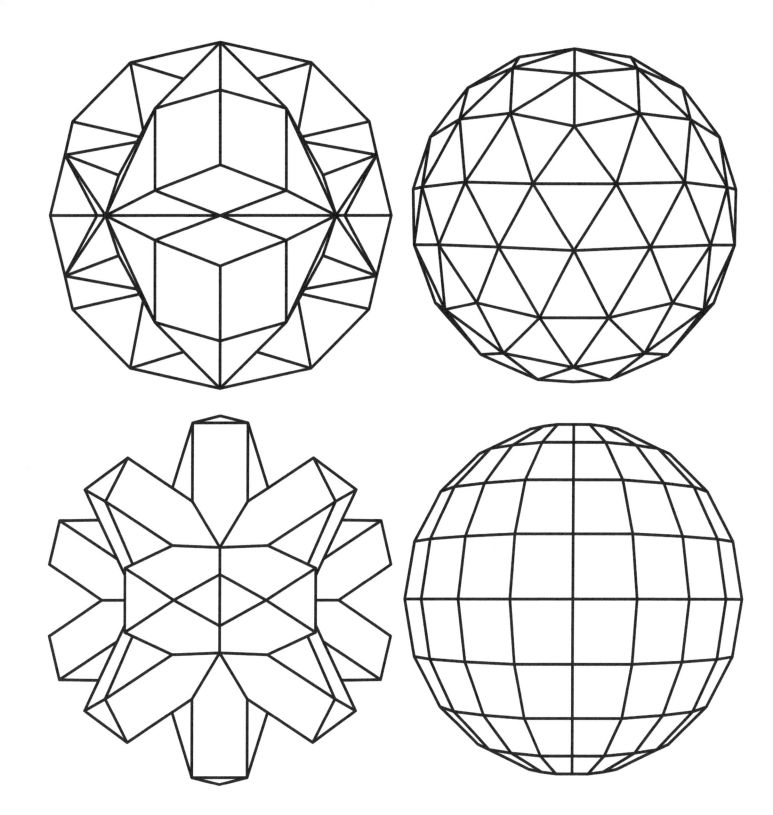

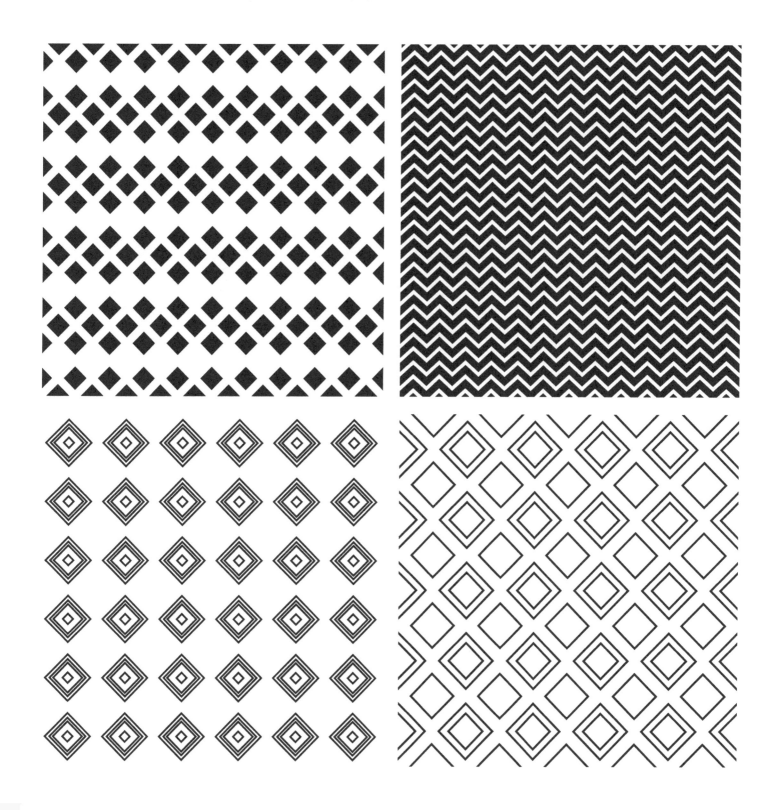

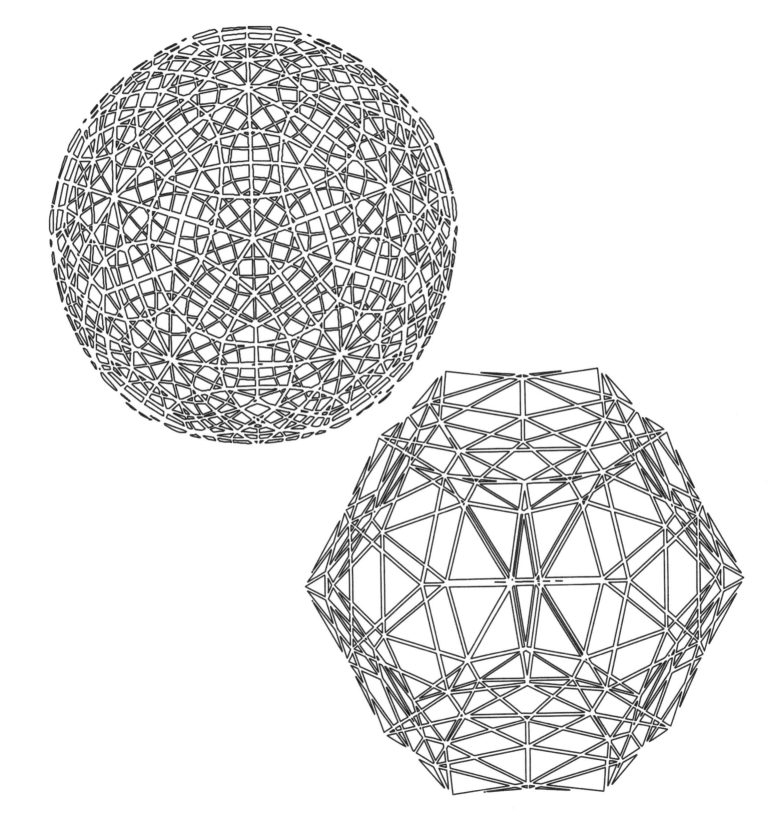

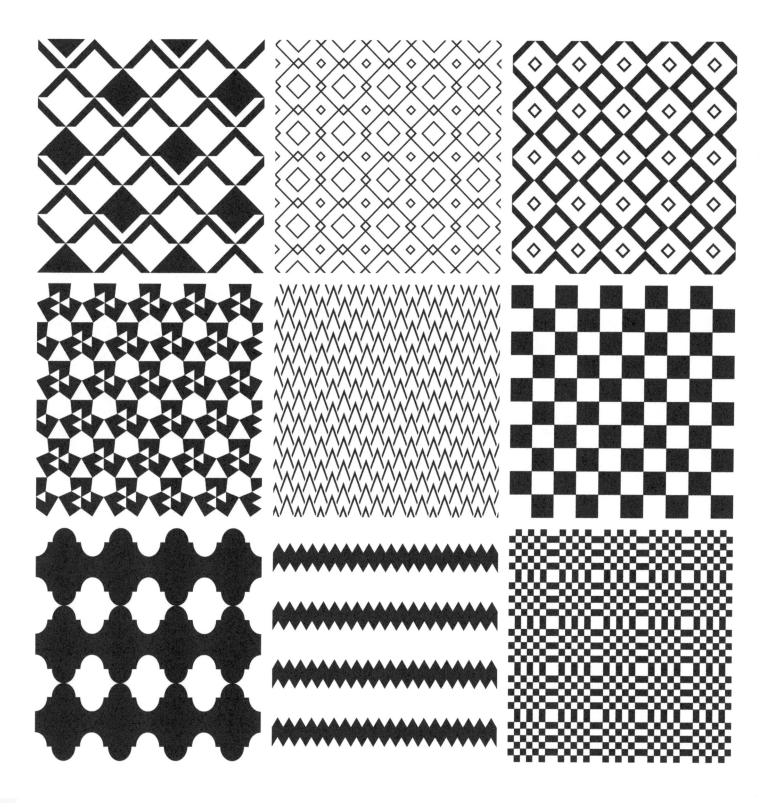

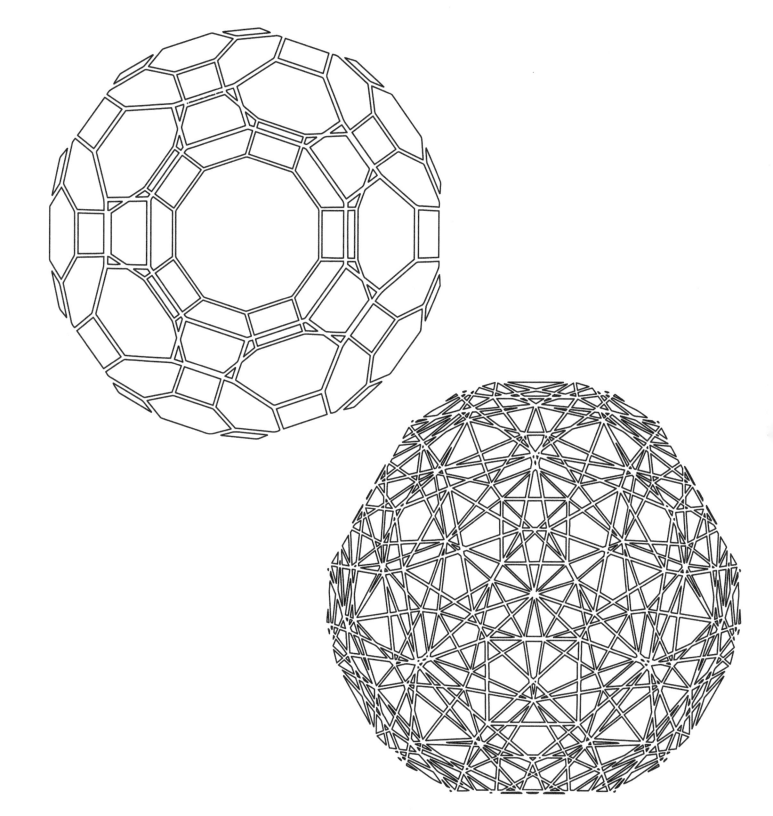

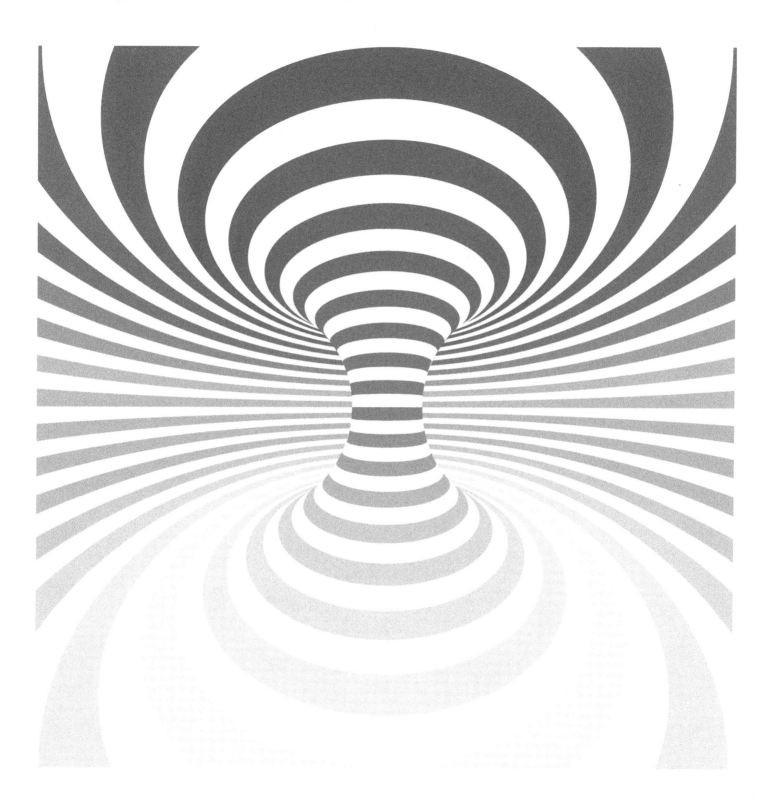

ART THERAPY COLORING BOOK SERIES

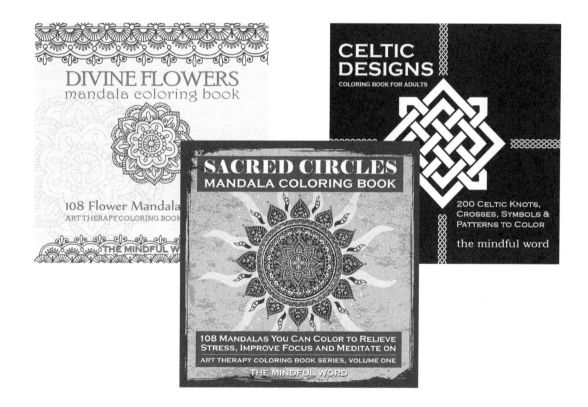

DIVINE FLOWERS
mandala coloring book
108 Flower Mandala
ART THERAPY COLORING BOOK
THE MINDFUL WORD

CELTIC DESIGNS
COLORING BOOK FOR ADULTS
200 CELTIC KNOTS, CROSSES, SYMBOLS & PATTERNS TO COLOR
the mindful word

SACRED CIRCLES
MANDALA COLORING BOOK
108 Mandalas You Can Color to Relieve Stress, Improve Focus and Meditate on
ART THERAPY COLORING BOOK SERIES, VOLUME ONE
THE MINDFUL WORD

www.themindfulword.org

CPSIA information can be obtained
at www.ICGtesting.com
Printed in the USA
LVHW102226041118
595948LV00015B/811/P

9 781987 869422